Geriatric Dental Medicine

Editors

JOSEPH M. CALABRESE
MICHELLE M. HENSHAW

CLINICS IN GERIATRIC MEDICINE

www.geriatric.theclinics.com

May 2023 • Volume 39 • Number 2

ELSEVIER

1600 John F. Kennedy Boulevard • Suite 1800 • Philadelphia, Pennsylvania, 19103-2899

http://www.theclinics.com

CLINICS IN GERIATRIC MEDICINE Volume 39, Number 2
May 2023 ISSN 0749–0690, ISBN-13: 978-0-443-18292-1

Editor: Taylor Hayes
Developmental Editor: Arlene Campos

Clinics in Geriatric Medicine (ISSN 0749-0690) is published quarterly by Elsevier Inc., 360 Park Avenue South, New York, NY 10010-1710. Months of issue are February, May, August, and November. Business and Editorial Offices: 1600 John F. Kennedy Blvd., Suite 1800, Philadelphia, PA 191023-2899. Periodicals postage paid at New York, NY, and additional mailing offices. Subscription prices are $312.00 per year (US individuals), $748.00 per year (US institutions), $100.00 per year (US & Canadian student/resident), $340.00 per year (Canadian individuals), $946.00 per year (Canadian institutions), $444.00 per year (international individuals), $946.00 per year (international institutions), and $195.00 per year (international student/resident). Foreign air speed delivery is included in all *Clinics* subscription prices. All prices are subject to change without notice. POSTMASTER: Send address changes to *Clinics in Geriatric Medicine,* Elsevier Health Sciences Division, Subscription Customer Service, 3251 Riverport Lane, Maryland Heights, MO 63043. **Telephone: 1-800-654-2452 (U.S. and Canada); 314-447-8871 (outside U.S. and Canada). Fax: 314-447-8029.** E-mail: journalscustomerservice-usa@elsevier.com **(for print support)** or journalsonlinesupport-usa@elsevier.com **(for online support).**

Reprints. For copies of 100 or more, of articles in this publication, please contact the Commercial Reprints Department, Elsevier Inc., 360 Park Avenue South, New York, New York 10010-1710. Tel.: 212-633-3874; Fax: 212-633-3820, E-mail: reprints@elsevier.com.

Clinics in Geriatric Medicine is covered in *MEDLINE/PubMed (Index Medicus), EMBASE/Excerpta Medica, Current Contents/Clinical Medicine (CC/CM),* and the *Cumulative Index to Nursing & Allied Health Literature.*

Contributors

EDITORS

JOSEPH M. CALABRESE, DMD
Associate Dean of Students, Director of Geriatric Dental Medicine, Clinical Professor, Department of General Dentistry, Boston University Henry M. Goldman School of Dental Medicine, Attending Dentist, Department of Medicine, Hebrew SeniorLife, Attending Dentist, Boston Medical Center, Boston, Massachusetts

MICHELLE M. HENSHAW, DDS, MPH
Associate Dean, Global and Population Health, Professor, Department of Health Policy and Health Services Research, Boston University Henry M. Goldman School of Dental Medicine, Boston, Massachusetts

AUTHORS

JOSEPH M. CALABRESE, DMD
Associate Dean of Students, Director of Geriatric Dental Medicine, Clinical Professor, Department of General Dentistry, Boston University Henry M. Goldman School of Dental Medicine, Attending Dentist, Department of Medicine, Hebrew SeniorLife, Attending Dentist, Boston Medical Center, Boston, Massachusetts

HELEN CHEN, MD
Chief Medical Officer, Hebrew SeniorLife, Assistant Professor of Medicine, Division of Gerontology, Beth Israel Deaconess Medical Center, Harvard Medical School, Boston, Massachusetts

RONALD ETTINGER, BDS, MDS, DDSc, DDSc(hc)
Professor Emeritus, Department of Prosthodontics, The University of Iowa College of Dentistry and Dental Clinics, Iowa City, Iowa

PAUL S. FARSAI, DMD, MPH
Clinical Professor, Department of General Dentistry, Boston University, Henry M. Goldman School of Dental Medicine, Boston, Massachusetts; Private Dental Practice, Swampscott, Massachusetts

ELISA M. GHEZZI, DDS, PhD
Adjunct Clinical Assistant Professor, University of Michigan School of Dentistry, South Lyon, Michigan

JENNIFER HARTSHORN, DDS
Clinical Associate Professor, Department of Preventive and Community Dentistry, The University of Iowa College of Dentistry and Dental Clinics, Iowa City, Iowa

MICHELLE M. HENSHAW, DDS, MPH
Associate Dean, Global and Population Health, Professor, Department of Health Policy and Health Services Research, Boston University Henry M. Goldman School of Dental Medicine, Boston, Massachusetts

JUDITH A. JONES, DDS, MPH, DScD
Professor, University of Detroit Mercy School of Dentistry, Detroit, Michigan

STEVEN KARPAS, DMD
Clinical Assistant Professor, Department of General Dentistry, Boston University Henry M. Goldman School of Dental Medicine, Boston, Massachusetts

MATTHEW MARA, DMD, EdM
Clinical Instructor, Department of General Dentistry, Boston University Henry M. Goldman School of Dental Medicine, Boston, Massachusetts

LEONARDO MARCHINI, DDS, MSD, PhD
Associate Professor, Department of Preventive and Community Dentistry, The University of Iowa College of Dentistry and Dental Clinics, Iowa City, Iowa

SARAH L. MEYER, MLIS
Assistant University Librarian, University of Florida Health Science Center Libraries, Gainesville, Florida

ROSEANN MULLIGAN, DDS, MS
Charles M. Goldstein Professor of Community Oral Health and Associate Dean, Community Health Programs and Hospital Affairs at the Herman Ostrow School of Dentistry of USC with a joint appoint at the Leonard Davis School of Gerontology of the University of Southern California, Los Angeles, California

LINDA C. NIESSEN, DMD, MPH, MPP
Dean and Professor, College of Dental Medicine, Vice Provost for Oral Health Affairs, Kansas City University of Medicine and Biosciences, Joplin, Missouri

KADAMBARI RAWAL, BDS, MSD, FASGD, FICD, FACD
Clinical Assistant Professor, Department of General Dentistry; Attending Dentist, Department of Medicine, Hebrew SeniorLife; Faculty Practice, Dental Health Center, Boston University Henry M. Goldman School of Dental Medicine, Boston, Massachusetts

FRANK A. SCANNAPIECO, DMD, PhD
Professor and Chair, Department of Oral Biology, School of Dental Medicine, University at Buffalo, The State University of New York, Buffalo, New York

ANNETTY P. SOTO, DMD
Clinical Assistant Professor, Division of General Dentistry, Department of Restorative Dental Sciences, University of Florida College of Dentistry, Gainesville, Florida

PIEDAD SUAREZ DURALL, DDS, MS
Associate Professor of Clinical Dentistry and Interim Division Chair, Dental Public Health and Pediatric Dentistry, Section Chair of Geriatrics and Special Patients, Director of the Special Patients Clinic of the Herman Ostrow School of Dentistry at USC, Adjunct Associate Professor, Leonard Davis School of Gerontology, University of Southern California, Los Angeles, California

LISA A. THOMPSON, DMD
Program Director, Geriatric Dental Fellowship, Harvard School of Dental Medicine, Boston, Massachusetts

Contents

The population of older adults is projected to increase dramatically as Baby Boomers continue to reach age 65 into 2029. This article discusses key shifts in this demographic, including changes in overall health status and living arrangements, that can aid in defining older adults and their medical needs. It also highlights the changes in dental use patterns and the increase in demand for comprehensive dental services for older adults in recent years. The article focuses on the fact that oral health contributes to overall health and the dental workforce must be prepared to treat older adults in their practices.

The number of individuals 65 and older living in the United States is increasing substantially and becoming more racially and ethnically diverse. This shift will affect the demographics of the patient population seeking dental care. It will also impact the future treatment needs of older adults. In older adults, similar to the general adult population, oral health disparities continue to exist related to race, ethnicity, gender, and socioeconomic level. Dental practitioners must understand these changes in order to meet the challenges of providing oral health care to the increasing numbers of diverse, medically compromised, and cognitively impaired older adults.

Most oral health care providers encounter older adults in their practices and can play a critical role in supporting independence and quality of life for this aging cohort. Physiologic and structural oral cavity changes associated with normal aging may affect the presentation and oral health care of older adults. This article reviews the normative aging of dentition and oral structures and physiologic changes associated with normal aging, including cardiovascular, metabolic, and musculoskeletal changes, and how they may affect oral health. Oral health providers should be aware of normal aging processes when they plan care or schedule procedures for older adults.

> Older adults have multiple morbidities that can impact oral, systemic, and psychological health. Although each disorder requires consideration from the provider before treatment, by assessing the common phenotypic presentations of older adults, we can better understand, select, and coordinate treatment modifications that would need to be considered and implemented for dental care.

> Aspiration pneumonia (AP), inflammation of the lung parenchyma initiated by aspirated microorganisms into the lower airways from proximal sites, including the oral cavity, is prevalent in, and problematic for, the elderly, especially those in institutions, and for those with several important risk factors. Many factors influence the pathogenesis of AP, including dysphagia, poor oral hygiene, diminished host defense, and underlying medical conditions. This article reviews the epidemiology, microbiology, pathogenesis, and prevention of AP, focusing on the role of poor oral health as a risk factor for, and on dental care for the prevention and management of, this important infection.

> Over the next several decades, rates of aged populations will increase rapidly. These populations are susceptible to multimorbidities and polypharmacy (concurrently, prescribed 5 or more medications). Many medications have side effects that manifest orally. Therefore, it essential to possess current pharmacologic knowledge to diagnose and treat oral implications of commonly prescribed medications. This article details common medication-induced oral lesions and patient assessment of risk factors for polypharmacy and provides a template to integrate medication reconciliation into dental clinical practice.

> Current research aims at improving early detection and treatment of cognitive impairment (CI), particularly in patients at high risk for progression to dementia. It is important to treat signs and symptoms as early as possible to normalize quality of life. In older cognitively impaired patients, dentists and physicians should consider polypharmacy, uncontrolled cardiovascular risk factors, depression, metabolic or endocrine derangements, delirium due to intercurrent illness, and dementia, all of which may increase risk for CI and other negative outcomes. An interdisciplinary team approach is a necessity for a responsible and safe treatment sequence.

When caring for the oral health of frail and functionally dependent older adults, it is important to understand their general health and oral health problems to make a diagnosis. There are multiple treatment strategies available to care for their needs; many may not be evidence based. Dental treatment planning for older adults is as much art as science and requires clinicians to understand how patients are functioning in their environments and how oral health care fits into their needs and lifestyle. This article discusses a variety of treatment planning techniques and illustrates the problem with a longitudinal case history.

Geriatric patients are more likely to have multiple medical comorbidities, physical limitations, and mental impairments that warrant careful consideration while providing patient care. Dentistry, along with other health care professional programs, incorporate interprofessional education (IPE) experiences to provide students with skills they need to deliver collaborative care in their future practice. Health professional programs should consider geriatric training in simulated learning environments, adult day programs, nursing homes, long-term care facilities, and home care experiences to provide students valuable IPE experiences. Lastly, this article presents a call to action for professional organizations to consider offering continuing education courses in IPE.

Older adults are retaining their teeth and need strategies for a lifetime of oral health care. Daily prevention and professional preventive care have the most significant impacts on reducing oral disease in the aging population. Providers of oral health care extend beyond traditional dental professionals to include caregivers and health care providers through teledentistry and interprofessional collaboration. Dental and aging organizations advocate for the inclusion of a dental benefit in Medicare to address access to care. Innovations in geriatric oral health care involve advances in clinical oral health care, delivery and models of care, funding, research, education, and policy.

CLINICS IN GERIATRIC MEDICINE

ISSUES OF RELATED INTEREST

Primary Care: Clinics in Office Practice
https://www.primarycare.theclinics.com/
Psychiatric Clinics
http://www.psych.theclinics.com/
Neurologic Clinics
http://www.neurologic.theclinics.com/

THE CLINICS ARE AVAILABLE ONLINE!
Access your subscription at:
www.theclinics.com

Preface

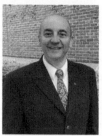 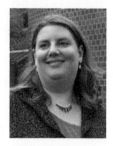

Joseph M. Calabrese, DMD   Michelle M. Henshaw, DDS, MPH
Editors

Welcome to the Geriatric Dental Medicine issue of *Clinics in Geriatric Medicine*. Given that older adults will become a greater percentage of your patients, we designed this issue to provide you with an overview of this special population's health and oral health needs as well as strategies to address these needs within your own practice and through referrals. This issue covers key concepts from demographic trends, to the challenges inherent in financing oral health care for older adults, to emerging technology. This issue also explores the value of working together as part of the health care team to reach the goal of delivering the highest-quality oral health care to older adults regardless of their complex medical status or if they are a long-term care resident. Even when that means making the difficult decision that the most appropriate treatment option is no treatment (do no harm).

The dental field has evolved from a "tooth fixer" to today where we play an integral role in the overall health and well-being of our patients as the dental medicine component of an interprofessional health care team. Throughout our careers in Geriatric Dental Medicine, we have worked alongside some of the most dedicated, thoughtful, and compassionate health care workers anywhere. We hope that this issue inspires you to expand your practice to include developing collaborations with nutritionists, physical therapists, occupational therapists, and other members of the health professions that can positively impact the health of your patients.

Ultimately, the quality of a product is due in large part to the sum of all its parts. We set the bar high and asked some of our esteemed colleagues to help author the 10 articles in this issue. We could not be more pleased with the results and feel that, in this case, the value of the issue as a whole exceeds the individual articles. We hope that you will find the information presented of great relevance and utility in your practice.

Clin Geriatr Med 39 (2023) ix–x
https://doi.org/10.1016/j.cger.2023.02.001
0749-0690/23/© 2023 Published by Elsevier Inc.

geriatric.theclinics.com

We would like to formally acknowledge the hard work and dedication of our contributing authors, and last, but not least, the outstanding team at Elsevier.

Joseph M. Calabrese, DMD
Boston University
Henry M. Goldman School of Dental Medicine
635 Albany Street, G-158
Boston, MA 02118-2308, USA

Michelle M. Henshaw, DDS, MPH
Boston University
Henry M. Goldman School of Dental Medicine
560 Harrison Avenue, Room 301
Boston, MA 02118, USA

E-mail addresses:
jobean@bu.edu (J.M. Calabrese)
mhenshaw@bu.edu (M.M. Henshaw)

Demographics and Oral Health Care Utilization for Older Adults

Joseph M. Calabrese, DMD[a,b,c],
Kadambari Rawal, BDS, MSD, FICD[b,d],*

KEYWORDS

- Older adult demographics • Dental service use • Oral health • Living arrangement
- Population trends • Dental care and demand

KEY POINTS

- In 2034, 1 in 4 Americans will be over the age of 65 and for the first time in US history there will be more older adults than people below the age of 18.
- A variety of social, cultural, economic, functional, and general vulnerability factors can aid in assessing the overall health status of older adult patients and determining the appropriate delivery of care for this demographic.
- Older adults are retaining their natural dentition for longer than previous generations and the need and use of comprehensive dental services is increasing.
- Disparities between dental use based on older adults' socioeconomic backgrounds are evident; policymakers should work on Medicaid and Medicare reforms to improve access to oral health care for all older adults.
- The integration of oral health and overall health would greatly benefit the older adult population.

DEFINITION OF OLDER ADULTS

According to the United Nations' 2019 report on World Population Aging, older persons are those 65 years of age or older.[1] Researchers continue to face challenges on how to integrate an appropriate multidimensional definition that incorporates chronologic, social, cultural and functional markers to help define the process of aging.[2] Although it is difficult to find a single comprehensive definition for old age, for several years,

This article originally appeared in Dental Clinics, Volume 65 Issue 2, April 2021.
[a] Department of General Dentistry, Student Affairs, Boston University Henry M. Goldman School of Dental Medicine, 635 Albany Street, Suite G158, Boston, MA 02118, USA;
[b] Department of Medicine, Hebrew SeniorLife, 1200 Centre Street, Boston, MA 02131, USA;
[c] Boston Medical Center, One Boston Medical Center Place, Boston, MA 02118, USA;
[d] Department of General Dentistry, Faculty Practice, Dental Health Center, Boston University Henry M. Goldman School of Dental Medicine
* Corresponding author.
E-mail address: kady@bu.edu

sociologists have divided older adults into 3 life-stage subgroups: the young-old (approximately 65–74 years), the middle-old (ages 75–84), and the old-old (over age 85).[3]

Over the past years, there has been an increased research interest on older adults. As a result of this, several previously used terms have been retired. **Box 1** illustrates an updated glossary of commonly used terms in geriatrics. Terms such as elderly (unless used to describe an entire population) are no longer used owing to their negative perpetuation of stereotypes (see **Box 1**). Another commonly used term that has recently been under much controversy and debate is "successful aging," the new definition emphasizes "being able to anticipate and cope with age related changes,"[5,6] rather than "freedom from disease and active engagement with life," as originally proposed by Rowe and Kahn in 1998.[7]

Based on their functional ability, older adults can be broadly classified as robust, frail, or dependent.[8] Frailty is defined as a "state of increased vulnerability to stressors owing to age related decline in physiologic reserve across neuromuscular, metabolic and immune systems."[9] Frail older adults have difficulties with instrumental activities of daily living (ADLs). Dependent older adults are those with difficulties with basic ADLs[10] (see **Box 1**). Older adults can be further classified based on their dependency.[10,11] **Table 1** has been reproduced from Federation Dentaire International's 2019 Roadmap for Healthy Aging.[10] It is a valuable model for application in a variety of scenarios, including policy development and treatment planning.[12,13]

Having considered recent developments in the definition of aging, the 2015 World Health Organization World report on Aging and Health made significant changes to their definition. They stated that, owing to the growing diversity in older populations, there is "no typical older person" and no standard age for retirement; globally, populations are becoming older with an improved survival beyond the age of 65 years.[14] According to the Gerontological Society of America's report in 2018, in the United States, the population of older adults is projected to exceed the population group younger than 18 years by 2035 (**Fig. 1**). It is predicted that a large numbers of Americans will continue to live in good health far past traditional retirement age.[15] The report emphasized that generalizations made about age-specific functional limitations have been proven incorrect and studies have shown that more than 50% of people who

---

Box 1
Glossary of terms

Older adults: Persons aged ≥65 years.[a]

Successful aging: A multidimensional concept, an ability of older adults to anticipate and cope with impending or existing age related changes.

Frailty: A state of increased vulnerability to stressors owing to age related decline in physiologic reserve across neuromuscular, metabolic and immune systems.

ADLs: A term used to collectively describe fundamental skills that are required to independently care for oneself such as eating, bathing, and mobility.[4]

Basic ADLs: Skills required to manage one's basic physical needs including personal hygiene or grooming, dressing, toileting, transferring or ambulating, and eating[4]

Instrumental ADLs: Include more complex activities that are related to the ability to live independently in the community. This would include activities such as managing finances and medications, food preparation, housekeeping, laundry.[4]

[a]CDC's Indicator definition for Older Adults; available at: https://www.cdc.gov/cdi/definitions/older-adults.html.*Abbreviation:* ADLs, Activities of Daily Living.

Table 1 Classification of older adults based on dependency/frailty[10]	
Level of Dependency	**Definition**
No dependency CSHA levels 1 and 2[12]	Robust people who exercise regularly and are the most fit group for their age.
Pre-dependency CSHA level 3	People with chronic systemic conditions that could impact oral health but, at the point of presentation, are not currently impacting oral health. A comorbidity whose symptoms are well controlled (4 in Pretty and colleagues[11]).
Low dependency CSHA level 4	People with identified chronic conditions that are affecting oral health but who currently receive or do not require help to access dental services or maintain oral health. These patients are not entirely dependent, but their disease symptoms are affecting them (4 in Pretty and colleagues[11]).
Medium dependency CSHA level 5	People with an identified chronic systemic condition that currently impacts their oral health and who receive or do not require help to access dental services or maintain oral health. This category includes patients who demand to be seen at home or who do not have transport to a dental clinic.
High dependency CSHA levels 6 and 7	People who have complex medical problems preventing them from moving to receive dental care at a dental clinic. They differ from patients categorized in medium dependency because they cannot be moved and must be seen at home.

Abbreviation: CSHA, Canadian Study of Health and Aging.

Roadmap for healthy ageing. Available at: https://www.fdiworlddental.org/sites/default/files/media/resources/ohap-2018-roadmap_ageing.pdf; with permission © FDI World Dental Federation 2018.

reach age 85 had no health-based limitations affecting their work or their housework (see **Fig. 1**).[16,17]

Hence, as the American and the global population continues to age, defying all previously set notions about old age, the definition of older adults remains fluid. Researchers must continue to acknowledge the diversity in aging and take into account a variety of factors, including social, cultural, economic, functional, and general vulnerability to assess the overall health status and the appropriate delivery of care for this demographic group.

CHANGES IN LIVING ARRANGEMENTS AND CONDITIONS

Several alterations associated with later life events can prompt a change in the living arrangements for older adults. These may include changes in the family structure, such as the loss of a spouse or partner, the onset of functional limitations, or changes in work and income such as retirement. Understanding the changes in living arrangements are paramount because these factors are important determinants of overall health and mortality of older adults.[18]

In 2012, the United States Aging Survey Findings revealed that, despite physical and economic difficulties, older Americans were determined to age in place.[19] Today,

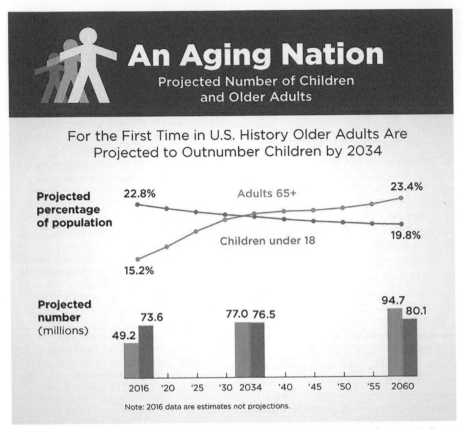

Fig. 1. Projected number of children and older adults in the United States. (*From* U.S. Census Bureau. National Population Projects, 2017. Available at: www.census.gov/programs-surveys/popproj.html.)

a majority of older Americans live in single-family homes, 76% are between 65 and 79 years of age, 68% are aged 80 years and over, and 26% live alone.[20] In 2006, 1 or more adult children lived approximately 280 miles from their older adult parent, but current research shows that multigenerational living arrangements are becoming more common.[21,22] Over the past decade, the percentage of older women living alone has decreased from 38% percent to 32%, although the percentage of older men living alone has increased slightly from 15% to 18%.[23]

In 2017, 59% of older adults lived with their spouse or partner and 11% of older adults lived with their adult children (with children moving into the parents' home or vice versa). The number of 3-generation households with at least 1 older adult family member increased to 3.2 million in 2016 from 1.7 million in 2006. Most of these 3-generation families were Hispanic and Asian households compared with other ethnic backgrounds. The 2018 report on Housing America's Older Adults showed that one-half of a million older adult households that include grandparents also had grandchildren but no middle generation present.[20]

With a larger older population aging in place, the demand for home health care services providing medical and other essential services is sure to increase. In 2006, 3 million Medicare beneficiaries received home health services, including skilled nursing, physical therapy, speech–language therapy, home aides, and medical social work. In 2007, it was estimated that 5% of older Americans received these services; models have predicted that by 2020 home health visits would increase by 36%.[24] The provision of these services enables older adults to maintain their autonomy and independence while receiving assistance with ADLs and instrumental ADLs in the comfort of their homes.

Assisted living facilities (ALFs) are becoming a more popular community living option available to those older adults who require assistance with ADLs. Many older Americans view ALFs as a home-like alternative to a wide range of long-term care facilities. Based on a social care model, they provide housing, meals, and assistance with ADLs, but are not intended to provide 24/7 skilled nursing care.[25] According to the National Center for Health Statistics: 2015-2016 report, more than 800,000 older Americans resided in ALFs as of 2014. The majority of these residents were categorized as 85 years and older, female, and non-Hispanic white.[26] Unlike long-term care facilities, ALFs do not come under federal regulations for staffing and training; smaller ALFs are private, for profit, and operate mainly through private funding, whereas larger ALFs may be part of larger chains and may accept Medicaid.[25]

In 2016, regulated long-term care service providers served more than 8.3 million Americans. These services included 4600 adult day services centers, 12,200 home health agencies, 4300 hospices, 15,600 nursing homes, and 28,900 assisted living and similar residential care communities (**Fig. 2**).[26]

Around 1.5 million older Americans (3.1%) aged 65 and over lived in institutional settings in 2016. Among them, 1.1 million lived in nursing homes. With increases in age, statisticians noted an increase in percentages among nursing home residents, ranging from 1% for those between 65 and 74 years of age to 3% for persons between the

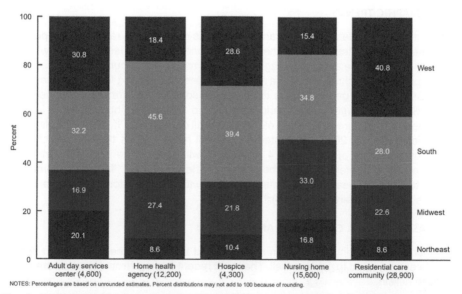

NOTES: Percentages are based on unrounded estimates. Percent distributions may not add to 100 because of rounding.

Fig. 2. Percent distribution of long-term care services providers, by sector and region: United States, 2016. (*From* National Center for Health Statistics. Long-term care providers and services users in the United States, 2015–2016. Available at: https://www.cdc.gov/nchs/data/series/sr_03/sr03_43-508.pdf. Accessed June 1, 2020.)

ages of 75 and 84 years of age, and 9% for those aged 85 years and older.[23] In 2018, the statistics changed, according to the Centers for Disease Control and Prevention (available at: www.cdc.gov/nchs/fastats/nursing-home-care.htm; www.cdc.gov/nchs/fastats/nursing-home-care.htm) 1.7 million people now reside in one of the 15,000 long-term care facilities around the United States in a given year.[26] For those seeking long-term care, 2 types of facilities are available. Skilled nursing facilities provide rehabilitative or postacute care immediately after an emergency hospital stay, whereas nursing homes and long-term care hospitals or long-term chronic care hospitals provide permanent custodial support, 24/7 medical care, along with assistance with ADLs. Unlike ALFs, nursing homes are mandated by federal regulations and usually accept Medicare and Medicaid.

Another model of care is the hospice and/or palliative care model that provides specialized medical care for older adults with chronic illnesses toward the end of life. This type of care can be delivered in the hospital, patient's home, nursing home, or as an outpatient at a doctor's office. In US hospitals with more than 50 beds, 25% reported a palliative care program in 2000, in 2016 that number increased to 75%.[27] Hospice care has a holistic and patient-centric approach, and these programs not only help older adults cope with their terminal illness, but they also provide support to their families. In 2017, there was a 4.7% increase in hospice care use by Medicare beneficiaries compared with the previous year and beneficiaries who identified as Asian and Hispanic have increased by 32% and 21%, respectively, since 2014. Sixty percent of hospice care recipients in 2017 were women and 66% were over the age of 80 years.[28] The demand for aging in place and hospice care have increased in recent years. In 2019, an article in the *New England Journal of Medicine* reported that, for the first time since the early twentieth century, the home has surpassed the hospital as the most common place of death for older adults in the United States.[29]

DEMOGRAPHIC TRENDS

The United States' demographic transformation is caused by a rapidly aging population. The United States follows in the path of Japan and countries in Europe where a majority of the people are over the age of 65; as a result, the population in these countries is projected to shrink within the next 3 decades. Decreasing fertility rates and the aging Baby Boomer generation are the major reasons for this dramatic change in the United States. Currently, older Americans make up 15% of the population, but in 2030 as all the Boomers turn 65 or older, older adults will comprise 21% of the population. It is projected that by 2060, the United States will have 3 times the number of older adults over the age of 85. One in 4 Americans will be over the age of 65 and one-half of a million centenarians will be added to the population. This development is bound to increase health care demands, along with the need for more home health and assisted living services (**Fig. 3**).[30]

INCREASING DENTAL CARE NEEDS AND DEMAND

As older adults continue to grow in numbers and live longer, their oral health needs have been projected to grow as well. The most recent findings from literature are summarized herein.

Removable and Fixed Prosthodontics

The aging population in the United States is experiencing less edentulism (**Fig. 4**),[31,32] but owing to the sheer increase in the number of older adults, the number of

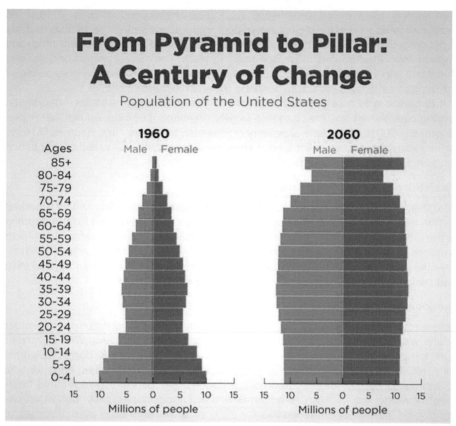

Fig. 3. US population by age and sex in 1960 compared with the US population projections in 2060. (*From* U.S. Census Bureau. National Population Projects, 2017. Available at: www. census.gov/programs-surveys/popproj.html.)

completely and partially edentulous arches are increasing. In 2013, iData Research Inc., performed a study showing that there were 2,822,589 complete dentures and 3,722,183 partial dentures fabricated for US patients, totaling 6,544,772; this change reflects an increase of 3.5% from the previous year.[33]

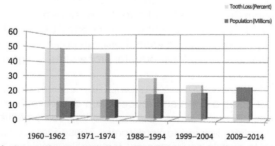

Fig. 4. Total population and prevalence of edentulism in U.S. adults (1960–2014). (*From* Dye, BA, Weatherspoon DJ, Lopez Mitnik G. Tooth loss among older adults according to poverty status in the United States from 1999 through 2004 and 2009 through 2014. J Am Dent Assoc. 2019;150(1):21; with permission. (Figure 3 in original).)

According to a dental prosthetics market analysis conducted in 2018,[34] an increased trend toward the digitization of dentures was evident. More dentists and patients were choosing digital dentures (both CAD/CAM and 3-dimensional printed) and implant-supported options to replace missing teeth. The market projections showed that fixed and removal partial dentures will continue to increase at the expense of full denture sales as older adults continue to retain more teeth.[31,34]

It is pertinent to note that, although overall the edentulous rates have decreased among older Americans the change is largely on account of older adults with higher incomes ($\geq$200% of the federal poverty guidelines), those with low incomes (<100% of the federal poverty guidelines) have shown a much smaller decrease in edentulous rates, highlighting the disparity within this demographic.[33]

Operative and Restorative Dental Procedures

A 2015 systematic review revealed that among global populations there was a marked shift in increased caries rates away from children and toward older adults. According to the article, caries rates peaked at age 70 likely owing to increased retention of teeth and loss of periodontal support, leading to an increased risk of root caries.[35] With increases in both coronal and root caries among older adults,[36] the need for operative and restorative dental procedures is expected to increase.

Endodontics

Often, root canal treatments become a necessity for tooth retention among older adults with systemic conditions that contraindicate tooth extraction. With advanced age, the pulpo–dentinal complex undergoes calcific changes that pose challenges for clinicians but with the advent of technologies such as microguided endodontics, an increased number of endodontists are successfully performing root canal treatments for older adults.[37] An American Board of Endodontics survey found that patients over the age of 65 accounted for 26% of all patients seen by diplomates of the board.[38] In the future, the need for root canal procedures will continue to increase in this cohort.

Periodontology

The current generation of older Americans have a greater number of teeth and implants than previous generations. With an uptick in the retention of natural dentition, there is an increase in both the prevalence and the incidence of periodontal disease among older adults.[39] Studies show that the cumulative nature of periodontal disease increases in severity as people age.[36] A 2015 study based on National Health and Nutrition Examination Survey data showed that the prevalence of periodontal disease steadily increases from 30 to 80 years of age.[40] This development compounded by limitations in manual dexterity and the inability to perform ADLs affects overall oral hygiene and can worsen underlying periodontal disease conditions among some older adults.[39] As such, the need to seek periodontal procedures is higher in this cohort.

Other Clinical Needs

One of the effects of aging on skin and mucosa is a decreased capacity for wound healing. An increase in medications and underlying comorbidities is known to decrease salivary function, leading to xerostomia. These factors, combined with an increased exposure to certain environmental factors like smoking, increase the risk of oral pathologies in older adults.[36]

Oral surgery options for the treatment of trauma, along with oral and oropharyngeal cancers, continue to be offered to older adults, but studies show that nonsurgical options or no treatment are commonly selected by older adults with increased age and late stage cancers.[41] Nonrestorable caries and nonrestorable fractured teeth commonly occur in these populations. Extractions are a common treatment modality chosen by older Americans belonging to low socioeconomic backgrounds and among medically compromised older adults toward the end of life.[42] Facial, especially nasal bone fractures are also common among older adults as a consequence of falls, and these fractures require treatment and often hospitalization as well.[43] Thus, the data shows that there is an increased need for oral maxillofacial surgery procedures.

Temporomandibular joint disorders are also common among older adults[44] owing to the degeneration of the surrounding muscles and disc. Pain management, physical therapy, and sometimes surgical intervention may be needed to adequately treat these conditions. According to a 2017 study, adults in their 60s and 70s showed some interest in receiving orthodontic treatment; their top reasons were maligned teeth, difficulty in chewing, and a need to improve esthetics. It is expected that an increasing number of older adults will opt for orthodontic treatment in the years to come.[45,46] Thus, orthodontic and orthognathic procedures are also becoming more common among this generation of older adults compared with previous generations.

These data show that the scope and need for all types of dental treatment among older adults is expanding. Oral health care providers may need to explore new interdisciplinary and collaborative approaches to meet the complex and rising needs of the "new" older adult.

Dental use

According to the Health Policy Institute's 2019 Annual Dental Industry Report, 43.3% of older adults had a general dental visit in 2016, this indicated a 38.3% increase since 2000.[47] The study showed that dental care use was influenced by multiple factors, such as dental benefits coverage, household income, perceived affordability, and overall health outcomes. Among those older adults who visited the dentist in 2016, 68.7% had private dental insurance and 37.5% were uninsured. Use rates were lowest (16.1%) among seniors with public dental coverage (Medicaid, Veterans Affairs, etc); 61.3% of older adults were high income ($\geq$400% of the federal poverty guidelines), whereas 24.4% were low income (<100% of the federal poverty guidelines). This disparity has increased since the early 2000s; higher income older adults are using dental services, whereas lower income older adults have shown no increase in use. The cost of care remains the number one barrier for use of dental services.[48] Although income- and race-related disparity barriers for dental service use are narrowing among US children, the trend among older adults is widening. This trend is problematic. Over the past few years, policymakers have been working on legislative reforms to bring dental care coverage to older Americans.[49] The expansion of dental benefits under Medicaid and introducing dental benefits in Medicare have also been proposed.[50]

In the past, studies on the use of dental services were focused mainly on community-dwelling older adults, but more recent studies have highlighted nursing home and hospitalized older adults as well.[51,52] The overall health of the geriatric patient was a significant predictor of dental care use in these studies. More studies of this kind are needed to motivate dentists to provide dental care for the vulnerable cohort residing in long-term care facilities.

A few years ago, many dentists believed that their dental education did not adequately prepare them to treat the older adult population and a small percentage of US dental schools offered clinical rotations (22.6%) in geriatric dental medicine.[53] Recent studies show a stark improvement in geriatric education. A higher percentage of dental schools now offer clinical rotations (57.1%) and mandatory courses in geriatric dental medicine.[54] The growth in geriatric dental education is necessary to prepare the dental workforce for the rising needs and use of dental services by older adults.

Oral health and overall health, a bidirectional relationship

The US Surgeon General's first report on Oral Health was released in 2000. The report stated that oral health is more than healthy teeth and is integral to the general health and well-being of all Americans, thus recognizing the impact of oral health on overall health.[55] Among older adults, oral health problems have long been identified as indicators of nutrition risk and involuntary weight loss. Strong associations exist between oral health and overall well-being[56] and oral health–related quality of life has important implications in the practice of geriatric medicine and research.[57]

Currently, more than 50% of older adults have 2 or more comorbid conditions (these include diabetes, dementia, depression, chronic obstructive pulmonary disease, cardiovascular disease, arthritis, and heart failure). As a result, they have greater health care needs and are subject to frequent hospitalizations and polypharmacy.[58] Oral health problems can occur in these older adults as either a cause or a consequence of various comorbidities and use of medications.[59]

An increase in the population of older adults is predicted to significantly burden the current health care system. Health care system reforms such as the development of collaborative care coordination models can help reduce this burden.[58] A 2005 paper drew attention to promoting the oral health of older adults through the Centers for Disease Control and Prevention's chronic disease model that is based on strong public health principles and population based approaches.[60] Dentists can play a significant role within these models as primary care providers or as part of a larger interdisciplinary health care team. This integration of oral health into overall health would greatly benefit the older adult population. Routine medical history evaluations before the dental appointment have shown to aid in the early identification and management of chronic disease risk factors.[61]

Several systemic disease conditions can be identified in the dental office during routine visits to the hygienist or the dentist. Oral manifestations of systemic disease include several autoimmune, hematologic, endocrine, neoplastic, and chronic disease conditions.[62] Similarly, some systemic diseases have been associated with oral infections.[63] The early identification of such infections can greatly minimize the immune burden on older adults especially those with multiple comorbidities. A 2019 systematic review also confirmed the evidence of an association between cognition and the oral health of older adults, encouraging the development of interventions focused on enhancing oral health outcomes for this cohort.[64]

In 2018, according to the Centers for Disease Control and Prevention more than one-half of the people living in the United States diagnosed with human immunodeficiency virus (HIV) were over the age of 50.[65] A growing number of older adults are now living with HIV; the average age of people with HIV is predicted to jump from 49 in 2015 to 58 in 2035 so the US HIV population will include a growing proportion of people 65 and older.[66] Research suggests that oral health care may improve the health-related quality of life of HIV/AIDS patients,[67] these findings reinforce that older adults with comorbidities, including those with HIV, deserve special attention to their health-related quality of life that includes oral care.

Thus, ample evidence exists to delineate the bidirectional relationship of oral health and systemic health in older adults. Medical and dental professionals should continue to collaborate and create patient-centric care delivery models to improve both systemic health and oral health outcomes for this demographic.

SUMMARY

The population of older adults is projected to increase dramatically as Baby Boomers continue to reach age 65 into 2029. In 2034, 1 in 4 Americans will be over the age of 65 and for the first time in US history there will be more older adults than people below the age of 18. As the American population continues to age, the definition of older adults remains fluid. Previously made generalizations about this demographic should be discarded. Health care providers and researchers should take into account a variety of factors including social, cultural, economic, functional, and general vulnerability to assess the overall health status of older adult patients and determine the appropriate delivery of care for this demographic. In a key shift from previous industry trends, a majority of this population now aspires to age in place. Most older Americans live in single-family homes, but multigenerational living arrangements are becoming more common. Although the number of assisted living and long-term care facilities are growing in the United States, research shows that the demand for aging in place and hospice care have increased in recent years. Oral health care providers must take this shift in living trends under consideration to develop the most effective treatment delivery options for this demographic.

With regard to oral health, older adults are retaining their natural dentition. There is an increase in caries risk and an increased need and demand for endodontic treatment, periodontal therapy, oral surgery procedures, and even orthodontic treatment among this cohort. The provision of comprehensive dental care is now common and made possible owing to the advent of technology. Oral health care providers should continue to create novel approaches and work in interdisciplinary collaborative teams to meet the complex oral health needs of this population. With increasing needs, the use of dental services is also on the rise, but so is the disparity between use patterns based on the socioeconomic status of older adults. The cost of care remains the number one barrier for use of dental services. The proposition of expanding dental benefits under Medicaid and introducing dental benefits in Medicare is promising and may help to resolve these issues.

A growth in geriatric dental education is evident from research, and this effort is necessary to prepare the dental workforce to meet the rising needs and use of dental services. Lastly, medical longevity has caused an increased burden of chronic disease conditions in the older adult population. Recognizing the association between oral health and overall health, medical and dental professionals should continue to collaborate and create patient centric care delivery models that improve health outcomes for this demographic.

CLINICS CARE POINTS

- In 2034, 1 in 4 Americans will be over the age of 65 and for the first time in US history there will be more older adults than people below the age of 18.
- The definition of older adults remains fluid owing to the growing diversity in older populations. There is no typical older person and no standard age for retirement.
- A variety of social, cultural, economic, functional, and general vulnerability factors can aid in assessing the overall health status of older adult patients and determining the appropriate delivery of care for this demographic.
- Older adults are retaining their natural dentition for longer than previous generations.
- The need for and use of comprehensive dental services is increasing among older adults.

- Disparities between dental use based on older adults' socioeconomic backgrounds are evident. Policymakers should continue to work on both Medicaid and Medicare reforms to improve access to oral health care for all older adults.
- The integration of oral health and overall health would greatly benefit the older adult population.

DISCLOSURE

The authors have nothing to disclose. This article has no commercial or financial conflicts of interest and has no external funding sources for all authors.

REFERENCES

1. Un.org. 2019. World population ageing 2019. [online]. Available at: https://www. un.org/en/development/desa/population/publications/pdf/ageing/WorldPopulation Ageing2019-10KeyMessages.pdf. Accessed June 1, 2020.
2. World Health Organization. Definition of an older or elderly person. Health Statistics and Health Information Systems; 2013. Available at: https://www.who.int/gho/ publications/world_health_statistics/EN_WHS2013_Full.pdf. Accessed June 1, 2020.
3. Little W. Chapter 13. Aging and the elderly. [online]. 2012. Available at: https:// opentextbc.ca/introductiontosociology/chapter/chapter13-aging-and-the-elderly. Accessed June 1, 2020.
4. Edemekong PF, Bomgaars DL, Sukumaran S, et al. Activities of daily living (ADLs) [updated 2020 Apr 12]. In: StatPearls [Internet]. Treasure Island (FL): StatPearls Publishing; 2020. Available at: https://www.ncbi.nlm.nih.gov/books/NBK470404/.
5. Kahana E, Kahana B, Lee JE. Proactive approaches to successful aging: one clear path through the forest. Gerontology 2014;60(5):466-74.
6. Martineau A, Plard M. Successful aging: analysis of the components of a gerontological paradigm. Successful aging ou vieillissement réussi: analyse d'un paradigme gérontologique. Geriatr Psychol Neuropsychiatr Vieil 2018;16(1):67-77.
7. Rowe J, Khan R. Successful aging. New York (NY): Pantheon; 1998.
8. Fukai K, Hori K, Benz C, et al. 2019. Available at: https://www.fdiworlddental.org/ sites/default/files/media/resources/2019-fdi_ohap-chairside_guide-en.pdf. Accessed June 1, 2020.
9. Walston J, Hadley EC, Ferrucci L, et al. Research agenda for frailty in older adults: toward a better understanding of physiology and etiology: summary from the American geriatrics society/national institute on aging research conference on frailty in older adults. J Am Geriatr Soc 2006;54(6):991-1001.
10. Fdiworlddental.org. 2018. Roadmap for healthy ageing. [online]. Available at: https://www.fdiworlddental.org/sites/default/files/media/resources/ohap-2018-roadmap_ageing.pdf. Accessed June 1, 2020.
11. Pretty I-A, Ellwood R-P, Lo E-C-M, et al. The Seattle care pathway for securing oral health in older patients. Gerodontology 2014;31(Suppl. 1):77-87.
12. CSHA refers to the "Canadian study of health and aging". Original article by Rockwood K, Song X, MacKnight Ch et al, A global clinical measure of fitness and frailty in elderly people. CMAJ 2005;173(5):489-95.
13. Hyde S, Dupuis V, Mariri B-P, et al. Prevention of tooth loss and dental pain for reducing the global burden of oral diseases. Int Dent J 2017;67(October 1):19-25.

14. WHO World report on ageing and health. Apps.who.int.. 2015. Available at: https://apps.who.int/iris/bitstream/handle/10665/186468/WHO_FWC_ALC_15.01_ eng.pdf?sequence=1. Accessed June 1, 2020.

15. Longevity economics. Geron.org. 2018. Available at: https://www.geron.org/ images/gsa/documents/gsa-longevity-economics-2018.pdf. Accessed June 1, 2020.

16. Bloom DE, Canning D, Fink G. Urbanization and the wealth of nations. Science 2008;319(5864):772–5.

17. Lowsky DJ, Olshansky SJ, Bhattacharya J, et al. Heterogeneity in healthy aging. J Gerontol A Biol Sci Med Sci 2014;69(6):640–9.

18. Russell D, Breaux E. Living arrangements in later life. In: Gu D, Dupre M, editors. Encyclopedia of gerontology and population aging. Cham (Switzerland): Springer; 2019.

19. The United States of aging survey national findings. Ncoa.org. 2012. Available at: https://www.ncoa.org/wp-content/uploads/8-3-12-US-of-Aging-Survey-Fact-Sheet-National-FINAL.pdf. Accessed June 1, 2020.

20. Housing America's older adults 2018. Jchs.harvard.edu. 2020. Available at: https://www.jchs.harvard.edu/sites/default/files/Harvard_JCHS_Housing_Americas_ Older_Adults_2018_1.pdf. Accessed June 1, 2020.

21. Profile of older Americans. Acl.gov. 2018. Available at: https://acl.gov/sites/ default/files/Aging%20and%20Disability%20in%20America/2018OlderAmericans Profile.pdf. Accessed June 1, 2020.

22. Caring for America's Seniors. Hcaoa.org. 2016. Available at: https://www.hcaoa. org/value-of-home-care.html. Accessed June 1, 2020.

23. Harris-Kojetin LSM, Lendon JP, Rome V, et al. Long-term care providers and services users in the United States, 2015–2016. National Center for Health Statistics; 2019.

24. Institute of Medicine (US). Committee on the future health care workforce for older Americans. Retooling for an aging America: building the health care workforce. 2, Health Status and Health Care Service Utilization. Washington (DC): National Academies Press (US); 2008. Available at: https://www.ncbi.nlm.nih.gov/books/ NBK215400/.

25. Han K, Trinkoff AM, Storr CL, et al. Variation across U.S. assisted living facilities: admissions, resident care needs, and staffing. J Nurs Scholarsh 2017;49(1): 24–32.

26. Long-term care providers and services users in the United States, 2013–2014. Cdc.gov. 2016. Available at: https://www.cdc.gov/nchs/data/series/sr_03/sr03_ 038.pdf. Accessed June 1, 2020.

27. Growth of palliative care in U.S. Hospitals: 2018 Snapshot (2000-2016). Media.-capc.org. 2018. Available at: https://www.capc.org/capc-reports-and-publications. Accessed June 1, 2020.

28. National hospice and palliative care organization report 2019. 39k5cm1a9u1968hg74aj3x51-wpengine.netdna-ssl.com. 2019. Available at: https://39k5cm1a9u1968hg74aj3x51-wpengine.netdna-ssl.com/wp-content/ uploads/2019/07/2018_NHPCO_Facts_Figures.pdf. Accessed June 1, 2020.

29. Cross SH, Warraich HJ. Changes in the place of death in the United States. N Engl J Med 2019;381(24):2369–70.

30. U.S. Census Bureau. National population projections tables: main series. 2017. Available at: https://www.census.gov/data/tables/2017/demo/popproj/2017-summary-tables.html. Accessed June 1, 2020.

31. Dye BA, Weatherspoon DJ, Lopez Mitnik G. Tooth loss among older adults according to poverty status in the United States from 1999 through 2004 and 2009 through 2014. J Am Dent Assoc 2019;150(1):9–23.

32. Albino J, Dye B, Ricks T. Surgeon general's report oral health in America: advances and challenges. Nidcr.nih.gov. 2020. Available at: https://www.nidcr.nih.gov/sites/default/files/2019-08/SurgeonGeneralsReport-2020_IADR_June%202019-508.pdf. Accessed June 1, 2020.

33. Gellar M, Alter D. The impact of dentures on the nutritional health of the elderly • jarlife. [online] Jarlife.net. 2020. Available at: https://www.jarlife.net/872-the-impact-of-dentures-on-the-nutritional-health-of-the-elderly.html. Accessed June 1, 2020.

34. Dental Prosthetics Market Analysis, T. Dental prosthetics market analysis, size, trends | global | 2018-2024 | medsuite. [online] iData research 2018. Available at: https://idataresearch.com/product/dental-prosthetics-market/. Accessed June 1, 2020.

35. Kassebaum NJ, Bernabe E, Dahiya M, et al. Global burden of untreated caries: a systematic review and metaregression. J Dent Res 2015;94:650–8.

36. Lamster IB, Asadourian L, Del Carmen T, et al. The aging mouth: differentiating normal aging from disease. Periodontol 2000 2016;72(1):96–107.

37. Johnstone M, Parashos P. Endodontics and the ageing patient. Aust Dent J 2015; 60(Suppl 1):20–7.

38. Goodis HE, Rossall JC, Kahn AJ. Endodontic status in older US adults. Report of a survey. JADA 2001;132:1525–30.

39. Darby I. Periodontal considerations in older individuals. Aust Dent J 2015; 60(Suppl 1):14–9.

40. Eke PI, Thornton-Evans GO, Wei L, et al. Periodontitis in US adults: National Health and Nutrition Examination Survey 2009-2014. J Am Dent Assoc 2018; 149(7):576–88.e6.

41. Goldenberg D, Mackley H, Koch W, et al. Age and stage as determinants of treatment for oral cavity and oropharyngeal cancers in the elderly. Oral Oncol 2014; 50(10):976–82.

42. Tiwari T, Scarbro S, Bryant LL, et al. Factors associated with tooth loss in older adults in rural Colorado. J Community Health 2016;41(3):476–81.

43. Marchini L, Allareddy V. Epidemiology of facial fractures among older adults: a retrospective analysis of a nationwide emergency department database. Dent Traumatol 2019;35(2):109–14.

44. Yadav S, Yang Y, Dutra EH, et al. Temporomandibular joint disorders in older adults. J Am Geriatr Soc 2018;66(6):1213–7.

45. Kim Y. Study on the perception of orthodontic treatment according to age: a questionnaire survey. Korean J Orthod 2017;47(4):215–21.

46. Pithon MM. Orthodontic treatment in an elderly patient with extraction of upper premolar. Gerodontology 2012;29(2):e1146–51.

47. Yarbrough C, Vujicic M. Oral health trends for older Americans. J Am Dent Assoc 2019;150(8):714–6.

48. Vujicic M, Buchmueller T, Klein R. Dental care presents the highest level of financial barriers, compared to other types of health care services. Health Aff (Millwood) 2016;35(12):2176–82.

49. Medicare Dental, Vision, and Hearing Benefit Act of 2019, HR 1393, 116th Cong. Available at: https://www.congress.gov/bill/116th-congress/house-bill/1393?q=%7B%22search%22%3A%5B%22HR+1393%22%5D%7D&s=1&r=1. Accessed June 3, 2020.

50. Center for Medicare Advocacy dental/oral health. Available at: https://www.medicareadvocacy.org/medicare-info/dental-coverage-under-medicare/. Accessed June 3, 2020.
51. Scannapieco FA, Amin S, Salme M, et al. Factors associated with utilization of dental services in a long-term care facility: a descriptive cross-sectional study. Spec Care Dentist 2017;37(2):78–84.
52. Rawal K, Sohn W, Calabrese J, et al. End of life dental service utilization by geriatric patients in a long-term care setting. [Master's dissertation] Boston University. 2018. Available at: https://hdl.handle.net/2144/32948. Accessed June 3, 2020.
53. Levy N, Goldblatt RS, Reisine S. Geriatrics education in U.S. dental schools: where do we stand, and what improvements should be made? J Dent Educ 2013;77(10):1270–85.
54. Ettinger RL, Goettsche ZS, Qian F. Predoctoral teaching of geriatric dentistry in U.S. dental schools. J Dent Educ 2017;81(8):921–8.
55. Hovland EJ. The surgeon general's report on oral health. LDA J 2000;59(4):13–4.
56. Bailey RL, Ledikwe JH, Smiciklas-Wright H, et al. Persistent oral health problems associated with comorbidity and impaired diet quality in older adults [published correction appears in J Am Diet Assoc. 2004 Oct;104(10):1548]. J Am Diet Assoc 2004;104(8):1273–6.
57. Porter J, Ntouva A, Read A, et al. The impact of oral health on the quality of life of nursing home residents. Health Qual Life Outcomes 2015;13:102.
58. Kastner M, Cardoso R, Lai Y, et al. Effectiveness of interventions for managing multiple high-burden chronic diseases in older adults: a systematic review and meta-analysis. CMAJ 2018;190(34):E1004–12.
59. Ghezzi EM, A J. Ship Systemic diseases and their treatments in the elderly: impact on oral health. J Public Health Dent 2000;60:289–96.
60. Gooch BF, Malvitz DM, Griffin SO, et al. Promoting the oral health of older adults through the chronic disease model: CDC's perspective on what we still need to know. J Dent Educ 2005;69(9):1058–63.
61. Douglass CW, Jiménez MC. Our current geriatric population: demographic and oral health care utilization. Dent Clin North Am 2014;58(4):717–28.
62. Gaddey HL. Oral manifestations of systemic disease. Gen Dent 2017;65(6):23–9.
63. Li X, Kolltveit KM, Tronstad L, et al. Systemic diseases caused by oral infection. Clin Microbiol Rev 2000;13(4):547–58.
64. Nangle MR, Riches J, Grainger SA, et al. Oral health and cognitive function in older adults: a systematic review. Gerontology 2019;65(6):659–72.
65. HIV and older Americans. cdc.gov. 2019. Available at: https://www.cdc.gov/hiv/group/age/olderamericans/index.html. Accessed October 12, 2020.
66. Smit M, Cassidy R, Hallett T. Quantifying the future clinical burden of an ageing HIV-positive population the USA: a mathematical modelling study. Glasgow (Scotland): HIV Drug Therapy; 2016 [Abstract P157].
67. da Costa Vieira V, Lins L, Sarmento VA, et al. Oral health and health-related quality of life in HIV patients. BMC Oral Health 2018;18(1):151.

Oral Health Disparities and Inequities in Older Adults

Michelle M. Henshaw, DDS, MPH[a],*, Steven Karpas, DMD[b]

KEYWORDS

• Oral health • Older adults • Disparities • Inequities • Dental caries
• Periodontal disease • Tooth loss • Oral cancer

KEY POINTS

• Oral health disparities exist in the US population and are among the most profound health disparities in the United States.

• As the US population ages and becomes more diverse, oral health disparities in older adults will likely increase. It is incumbent upon dental professionals to recognize the distribution of oral disease in all older adult subpopulations and how this impacts clinical care.

• As the population of older adults continues to become more racially and ethnically diverse, it can be expected that both the percentage and the absolute numbers of older adults with dental treatment needs will increase.

• Older adults are more likely to be dentally uninsured/underinsured, are less likely to receive timely care, and therefore, are more likely to have untreated disease become symptomatic.

• In order to eliminate oral health disparities in older adults, the dental profession must develop and ensure access to culturally appropriate clinical care and health policies that foster tooth retention and the successful maintenance of good oral health in all populations of older adults.

INTRODUCTION

In all populations, good oral health is essential to overall health and well-being; however, this is especially true in older adults.[1] Despite improvements in the oral health status of the US population as a whole, not all groups have benefited from these improvements equally. A disproportionately higher burden of oral diseases and disorders is still borne by certain population groups, including patients with special needs, older

The authors have no conflicts of interest to disclose.
This article originally appeared in Dental Clinics, Volume 65 Issue 2, April 2021.
[a] Department of Health Policy and Health Services Research, Boston University Henry M. Goldman School of Dental Medicine, 560 Harrison Avenue, Suite 301, Boston, MA 02118, USA;
[b] Department of General Dentistry, Boston University Henry M. Goldman School of Dental Medicine, 635 Albany Street, Boston, MA 02118, USA
* Corresponding author.
E-mail address: mhenshaw@bu.edu

adults, minorities, and individuals with low income.[2–4] The differences in health status, health outcomes, or health care use between distinct groups are known as health disparities. There are many definitions of health disparities, including the one used by Healthy People:[3]

"... a particular type of health difference that is closely linked with social, economic, social, and/or environmental disadvantage. Health disparities adversely affect groups of people who have systematically experienced greater obstacles to health based on their racial or ethnic group; religion; socioeconomic status; gender; age; mental health; cognitive, sensory, or physical disability; sexual orientation or gender identity; geographic location; or other characteristics historically linked to discrimination or exclusion."

Although the Healthy People definition of health disparities links group differences to a disadvantage, by the strictest definition, a health disparity can be any difference in health status. In contrast, health inequities, a term used more commonly than health disparities in other countries and increasingly being used in the United States, are health differences that are avoidable, unnecessary, and unjust.[4] Of course, not all health differences are avoidable, such as prostate cancer in men versus women, or unjust, such as the proportion of hockey players who have had fractured teeth compared with the general population. It is, however, unjust if individuals are unable to attain health or are denied quality health care because they belong to a particular group.[5] It can also be said that equal treatment may still be unjust if some disadvantaged groups need and do not receive more resources or services than others to be healthy.[6] A related concept, social justice, purports that everyone deserves equal rights and opportunities[7] and often can be most effectively achieved by addressing systemic level factors, as seen in **Fig. 1**.[8] For example, an older adult with arthritis may need an adaptive aid in order to use their toothbrush, a resource not needed by an individual without arthritis, and a low-income elder at highest risk for oral disease who would benefit the most from brushing may not be able to afford a toothbrush at all. Making toothbrushes a Medicare benefit could provide everyone equal access to toothbrushes.

The factors contributing to health disparities and inequities are complex. When exploring the root causes of health inequities, the importance of the social determinants of health is clear. Social determinants of health are "the conditions in which people are born, grow, work, live, and age, and the wider set of forces and systems shaping the conditions of daily life. These forces and systems include economic

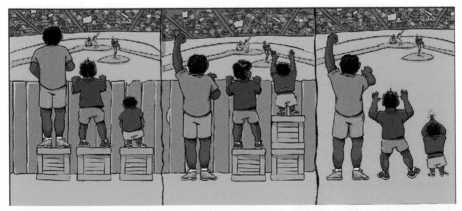

Fig. 1. Equality, equity, and social justice. (*Adapted from* Interaction Institute for Social Change | Artist: Angus Maguire; with permission.)

policies and systems, development agendas, social norms, social policies and political systems."[9] For example, access to dental care is influenced by public policies, insurance coverage, provider availability, transportation, ability to take time off from work, cultural norms, and perceived need. Other factors, such as bias, prejudice, discrimination, and stereotyping, at the provider, patient, institutional, and health system level, contribute to disparities in quality of care, which then translate into health disparities. The contribution of biology to health disparities has also been explored. For example, chronic stress experienced disproportionately by individuals with lower incomes can depress immune systems, activate inflammatory mediators, and shorten telomeres, all of which negatively impacts health.[6] These factors exist at the individual, family, and community levels,[10,11] and their multifaceted interplay contributes to the challenges both in understanding their relative contributions to oral health disparities and in developing effective models to prevent diseases.[12]

Disparities in oral health conditions are among the most profound health disparities in the United States.[2] As the US population ages and becomes more diverse, it is incumbent upon dental professionals to recognize the distribution of oral disease in all older adult subpopulations and the factors that put vulnerable populations at increased risk for oral disease. Understanding these factors is particularly challenging because older adults often have additional risk factors, such as comorbid conditions, pharmacotherapy, functional disabilities, and/or cognitive impairments, that may hamper daily oral hygiene care and the ability to access regular dental care. Older adults who receive regular dental care are more likely to have decayed teeth diagnosed and treated before experiencing pain and other symptoms. However, older adults, their families, and even health care providers may not perceive that oral health care and dental visits are important, especially when the older adult is edentulous or has complex medical issues.[13] Unfortunately, because in the United States insurance is tied to employment and Medicare does not cover routine dental care, older adults are also more likely to be dentally uninsured and underinsured, creating another barrier to dental care and exacerbating oral health disparities.[14]

When looking at the oral health disparities in US older adult subpopulations, poor individuals almost universally experience a greater burden of oral diseases and conditions than those with more resources.[15] Individuals from racial and ethnic minority groups, particularly blacks and Hispanics, also generally experience higher levels of untreated decay, periodontal disease, tooth loss, orofacial pain as well as higher oral cancer mortalities than non-Hispanic whites.[16] Data about tooth loss, dental caries, periodontal disease, and oral and pharyngeal cancer are generally measured to track oral health status at the population level. This information is measured by structured oral examinations as part of the ongoing National Health and Nutrition Examination Survey (NHANES). NHANES is a series of studies that combines interview and physical examinations to assess the health and nutritional status of community-dwelling adults and children in the United States, thereby producing health statistics for the nation. The initiative began in the 1960s and is now an on-going program of the Centers for Disease Control and Prevention. Each year, the survey examines a sample of about 5000 individuals that are representative of the general US population. The interview comprises demographic, socioeconomic, dietary, and health-related questions. The examination includes medical, dental, physiologic measurements, and laboratory tests.[17] NHANES data are stratified by age, race and ethnicity, poverty level, and gender, making it ideal data to assess health disparities in the United States. In the next few sections, NHANES data are used to provide information about the unequal distribution of the major oral diseases and conditions in the elder population: dental caries, periodontal disease, and tooth loss in the United States. Information about oral cancer comes primarily from the Surveillance, Epidemiology, and End Results Program of the National Cancer Institute.[18]

Dental Caries

Caries experience

To understand the extent of oral health disparities in older adults, reviewing the oral health status of younger adults as a reference can be useful. Of all dentate adults aged 20 to 64, 90% exhibited dental caries experience (either treated or untreated), and 27% had untreated decay.[19] Not surprisingly, dental caries experience was even greater in dentate adults 65 and older, with almost all of those examined (96%) having had caries experience. Within the older adult population, there was no difference when comparing caries experience in those 65 to 74 years of age to those greater than 75 years of age. What is surprising is that in contrast to the adult population less than 65 years of age in which caries experience decreased from 1999 to 2004 to 2011 to 2016, the prevalence in older adults increased by 3% during that same timeframe.[19]

Although there were no age disparities within the older adult population, racial and ethnic disparities existed. The prevalence of caries experience was higher among non-Hispanic white older adults compared with older non-Hispanic black and Hispanic adults. However, non-Hispanic blacks showed the largest increase in caries experience over time. Disparities in education level, income, and smoking status were also seen, with those with higher income, more education, and never smokers having more caries experience than those with lower income, less education, and a history of smoking[19] (**Table 1**). Unfortunately, trends in caries experience prevalence indicate the most vulnerable older adults in each category demonstrated a 3% to 5% point increase over time, and none had a statistically significant decrease. The exception was that caries prevalence in current smokers saw essentially no change.[19]

Untreated tooth decay

According to the NHANES data collected from 2011 to 2016, 16% of adults aged 65 and older had untreated tooth decay. Similar to caries experience, there were disparities in the prevalence of untreated decay based on race/ethnicity, income, education, and smoking status; however, the patterns of the disparities are different. Although the percentage of untreated decay in older adults was less than in the younger adult population, the relative differences in the subpopulations were larger,[19] meaning that subpopulations of older adults experience higher levels of disparities in untreated caries as compared with adults less than 65 years of age. In fact, older adults who were non-Hispanic black, Mexican American, poor, near poor, or current smokers had about 2 to 3 times the prevalence of untreated decay compared with those who had never smoked or were non-Hispanic white or not poor[19] (**Table 2**). It is important to note that there was a nonsignificant decrease in the prevalence of older adults with untreated decay compared with NHANES data collected in 1999 to 2004. However, 1 in 6 dentate older adults or 7.9 million people are estimated to have untreated decay.[19] Because this population continues to become more racially and ethnically diverse, given the significantly higher prevalence of untreated decay in non-Hispanic blacks and Mexican Americans, it can be expected that both this percentage and absolute numbers of older adults with dental caries will increase.

Periodontal Disease

Like dental caries, periodontal disease is not distributed evenly among the US adult population. Almost half (42%) of the US population older than 30 years of age was

Table 1
Prevalence of dental caries experience[a] among dentate adults aged 65 y or older, by selected characteristics, United States, National Health and Nutrition Examination Survey, 1999 to 2004 and 2011 to 2016

Characteristic	1999–2004		2011–2016		Change, %[c]
	%	SE	%	SE	
Total	93.0	0.64	96.2	0.51	3.2[d]
Age (y)					
65–74[b]	93.2	0.80	96.4	0.65	3.2
≥75	92.7	0.90	96.0	0.65	3.3[d]
Sex					
Male[b]	93.6	0.90	96.1	0.67	2.5[d]
Female	92.5	0.82	96.3	0.62	3.9[d]
Race and ethnicity					
White, non-Hispanic[b]	94.8	0.72	98.2	0.44	3.4[d]
Black, non-Hispanic	79.8	2.98	85.7[d]	1.93	5.9
Mexican American	84.1	1.83	85.3[d]	2.86	1.2
Poverty status					
<100% FPL	83.7	2.49	88.1[d]	2.17	4.4
100% to 199% FPL	90.9	1.38	94.0[d]	0.99	3.1
≥200% FPL[b]	95.5	0.70	98.2	0.43	2.7[d]
Poverty status					
<200% FPL	89.1	1.13	92.4[d]	1.10	3.3[d]
≥200% FPL[b]	95.5	0.70	98.2	0.43	2.7[d]
Education					
< High school	83.8	1.60	89.1[d]	1.52	5.3[d]
High school	94.3	1.24	95.3[d]	1.09	1.1
> High school[b]	97.2	0.63	98.3	0.33	1.1
Cigarette smoking history					
Current smoker	89.6	2.46	89.8[d]	2.66	0.1
Former smoker	93.5	0.95	96.2	0.79	2.8[d]
Never smoked[b]	93.0	0.90	96.8	0.57	3.8[d]

Note: All estimates are adjusted by age (5-y groups; maximum age group is >80) to the US 2000 standard population.

Abbreviations: FPL, federal poverty level; less than 100% FPL = poor; 100%–199% FPL = near poor; less than 200% FPL = poor and near poor combined; and ≥200% FPL = not poor; SE, standard error.

[a] Defined as having 1 or more untreated decayed or filled permanent teeth among adults with at least 1 permanent tooth.

[b] Reference group for comparisons within each characteristic, 2011 to 2016.

[c] Change in percentage points from 1999 to 2004 to 2011 to 2016. Positive value = increase; negative value = decrease.

[d] $P < .05$ based on t test for differences between 2 periods or 2 groups within each characteristic.

From Centers for Disease Control and Prevention. Oral Health Surveillance Report: Trends in Dental Caries and Sealants, Tooth Retention, and Edentulism, United States, 1999–2004 to 2011–2016. Atlanta, GA: Centers for Disease Control and Prevention, US Dept of Health and Human Services; 2019; with permission.

Table 2
Prevalence of untreated tooth decay in permanent teeth[a] among dentate adults aged 65 y or older, by selected characteristics, United States, National Health and Nutrition Examination Survey, 1999 to 2004 and 2011 to 2016

Characteristic	1999–2004		2011–2016		Change, %[b]
	%	SE	%	SE	
Total	18.1	1.01	15.9	1.20	−2.2
Age (y)					
65–74[c]	17.0	1.37	15.4	1.55	−1.6
≥75	19.5	1.28	16.5	1.40	−3.0
Sex					
Male[c]	20.4	1.34	18.0	1.53	−2.4
Female	16.4	1.18	14.2[d]	1.25	−2.3
Race and ethnicity					
White, non-Hispanic[c]	15.8	1.24	13.4	1.25	−2.4
Black, non-Hispanic	37.1	3.48	29.1[d]	2.49	−8.0
Mexican American	42.1	3.07	35.9[d]	3.24	−6.2
Poverty status					
<100% FPL	33.4	3.42	33.1[d]	3.18	−0.3
100% to 199% FPL	23.8	1.75	26.9[d]	2.64	3.1
≥200% FPL[c]	14.2	1.20	9.9	1.27	−4.3[d]
Poverty status					
<200% FPL	26.2	1.75	28.6[d]	2.30	2.4
≥200% FPL[c]	14.2	1.20	9.9	1.27	−4.3[d]
Education					
< High school	26.2	2.33	30.8[d]	2.76	4.7
High school	17.7	1.39	18.8[d]	2.22	1.1
> High school[c]	14.2	1.27	11.7	1.35	−2.5
Cigarette smoking history					
Current smoker	27.6	3.66	33.9[d]	5.10	6.3
Former smoker	18.6	1.31	15.3	1.67	−3.3
Never smoked[c]	16.5	1.30	14.2	1.37	−2.4

Note: All estimates are adjusted by age (5-y groups; maximum age group is ≥80) to the US 2000 standard population.

Abbreviations: FPL, federal poverty level; less than 100% FPL = poor; 100% to 199% FPL = near poor; less than 200% FPL = poor and near poor combined; and ≥200% FPL = not poor; SE, standard error.

[a] Defined as having 1 or more untreated decayed permanent teeth among adults with at least 1 permanent tooth.

[b] Change in percentage points from 1999 to 2004 to 2011 to 2016. Positive value = increase; negative value = decrease.

[c] Reference group for comparisons within each characteristic, 2011 to 2016.

[d] $P < .05$ based on *t* test for differences between 2 periods or 2 groups within each characteristic.

From Centers for Disease Control and Prevention. Oral Health Surveillance Report: Trends in Dental Caries and Sealants, Tooth Retention, and Edentulism, United States, 1999–2004 to 2011–2016. Atlanta, GA: Centers for Disease Control and Prevention, US Dept of Health and Human Services; 2019; with permission.

afflicted with periodontal disease as measured by NHANES data collected from 2009 to 2014,[20] using the Centers for Disease Control and Prevention/American Association of Periodontology case definitions for surveillance of periodontitis.[21,22] Because of the cumulative nature of periodontal disease, it is not surprising that the percentage of the population having periodontal disease increased with age. Those aged 30 to 44 had the lowest percentage of periodontal disease (29.5%), followed by those 45 to 64 years old (46%), and those 65 and older had the largest percentage (59.8%). In addition to these age disparities, there was a gender disparity, with a larger percentage of men having disease (50.2%) than women (34.6%).[20]

There was also disparity in racial/ethnic distribution of periodontitis. Hispanic populations experienced the highest prevalence of periodontal disease. In older adults, 79.4% of Mexican Americans had periodontal disease, compared with 72.6% of non-Hispanic blacks and only 56.3% of non-Hispanic whites.[20] Periodontitis was more common among those with lower educational attainment and income. Disparities also existed in health conditions and behaviors. Periodontal disease prevalence increased with smoking status, self-reported diabetes diagnosis, number of missing teeth, not using dental floss, and infrequent dental visits.[20] Similar trends were seen when considering only severe periodontal disease; there was a 3 times greater prevalence of severe periodontal disease in Mexican Americans, non-Hispanic blacks, and current smokers. However, there was not a statistically significant increase in periodontal disease prevalence with higher body mass index[20] (**Table 3**).

When analyzing the percentage of periodontal disease by severity levels among the total adult population, 34.4% had either mild or moderate cases of periodontitis, whereas 7.8% had severe periodontal disease.[22] The percentage of individuals with severe periodontal disease was lowest in those aged 30 to 44, but in those 45 and older, the prevalence remained relatively stable as age increased. In fact, the highest prevalence of severe periodontal disease was not seen in older adults (9.0%), but instead those aged 45 to 64 (10.4%).[20] Although the prevalence of mild and severe periodontitis increased slightly with age, the prevalence of moderate periodontitis significantly increased with age. This increase in prevalence of moderate periodontal disease was the driving factor in the increase in total periodontal disease diagnosis increasing with age[20] (**Fig. 2**).

The increasing prevalence of moderate periodontal disease, coupled with the increasing numbers of older adults in the subpopulations that have the highest rates of periodontal disease, suggests that there will be increased demand for preventive and treatment plans. Treatments will require tailoring to the periodontal risk and unique needs of their older adult patients after careful assessment of medical and social histories as well as physical and cognitive function.

Tooth Loss

Complete tooth loss is an oral health status indicator that has improved dramatically over time, and it is now largely a condition of older adults. Even within the population of adults 65 to 74 years old, complete tooth loss has decreased by more than 75% over the past 5 decades.[23] Consistent with this trend, when looking at the newest data from older adults, complete edentulism decreased from 27% to 17% from 1999 to 2004 to 2011 to 2016,[24] which means that 5 out of 6 older adults are at least partially dentate and will need dental restorative and periodontal treatment. Again, there were disparities by age. The percentage of edentulous individuals aged 65 to 74 years old decreased by almost 50% to 13% and those 75 years or older only decreased by 28% to 22.5%.[24] It is important to note that although there was a decrease in edentulism when looking only at age, that is only part of the picture. There were significant

Table 3 Prevalence of total (mild, moderate, or severe) periodontitis among dentate adults 30 y or older according to age group and demographic and health-related subgroups, National Health and Examination Survey 2009 to 2014 (N = 10,683)			
	Age Group, y, % (Standard Error)		
Characteristic	30–44	45–64	65 or Older
Total	29.4 (1.5)	46.0 (1.6)	59.8 (2.1)
Gender			
Male	37.5 (2.1)†	55.0 (1.5)†	66.6 (2.3)†
Female	21.5 (1.3)	37.4 (2.0)	53.8 (2.7)
Race/ethnicity			
Mexican American	52.2 (1.9)†	67.1 (3.0)†	79.4 (4.4)‡
Other Hispanic	40.9 (2.1)†	52.0 (2.4)‡	71.0 (4.1)§
Non-Hispanic white	20.7 (1.9)	40.0 (1.9)	56.3 (2.5)
Non-Hispanic black	42.7 (2.9)†	64.6 (2.0)†	72.6 (2.5)†
Other race, including multiracial	30.6 (2.1)†	54.5 (3.6)†	73.8 (5.5)§
Smoking status			
Nonsmoker	23.8 (1.6)	36.0 (1.8)	55.9 (2.5)
Former smoker	26.3 (2.3)	47.4 (2.5†)	61.2 (2.5)§
Current smoker	47.8 (2.5)†	74.3 (2.0)†	81.0 (4.2)†
Socioeconomic level			
<100% FPL#	50.7 (2.3)†	68.9 (2.1)†	70.0 (3.4)†
100% to 199% FPL	38.9 (2.2)†	62.2 (2.8)†	66.3 (3.0)†
200% to 399% FPL	26.5 (2.3)†	52.2 (2.7)†	63.6 (3.0)†
>400% FPL	15.0 (1.7)	30.8 (1.6)	49.5 (2.4)
Body mass index**			
<25	23.8 (1.8)	43.6 (2.6)	61.9 (3.1)
25–30	28.4 (1.8)§	46.1 (2.0)	58.9 (2.3)
>30	34.8 (2.0)†	47.3 (1.7)	58.6 (3.1)
Diabetes mellitus			
Yes	50.0 (5.2)†	56.8 (3.0)†	68.4 (3.3)‡
No	28.7 (1.5)	44.7 (1.6)	57.7 (2.2)
Use of dental floss in past 7 d			
Yes	26.1 (1.6)	40.1 (1.7)	56.7 (2.2)
No	37.4 (2.4)†	62.6 (1.9)†	67.0 (3.0)‡
No. of teeth missing			
0	20.2 (1.6)	25.2 (2.2)	37.9 (4.1)
1–5	33.9 (1.8)†	45.1 (1.7)†	56.7 (2.7)†
6–27	55.7 (2.4)†	71.9 (1.5)†	70.1 (2.1)†
Last dental visit, mo			

(continued on next page)

Table 3 *(continued)*			
	Age Group, y, % (Standard Error)		
Characteristic	30–44	45–64	65 or Older
≤6	16.9 (1.9)	30.1 (1.8)	49.2 (3.0)
6–12	24.5 (2.5)§	42.5 (3.2)†	60.1 (6.3)
>12 or never	42.5 (2.3)†	63.8 (2.2)†	68.9 (3.4)†

**Third molars were excluded. c2 and Wald F tests were used for testing significance of proportion and average, respectively, according to age group.
† NS: Not significant.
‡ Income values were missing in 895 respondents.
§ FPL: Federal poverty level. {Body mass index values in kilograms per square meter were missing in 64 respondents.
\# Based on data from the National Health and Nutrition Examination Survey 2011-2014 only.
From Eke PI, Thornton-Evans GO, Wei L, Borgnakke WS, Dye BA, Genco RJ. Periodontitis in US Adults: National Health and Nutrition Examination Survey 2009-2014. J Am Dent Assoc. 2018 Jul;149(7):576-588.e6. https://doi.org/10.1016/j.adaj.2018.04.023. PMID: 29957185; with permission.

disparities, notably a threefold increase in the prevalence of edentulism in older adults who were poor, had less than a high school education, or were current smokers compared with older adults who were not poor, had more than a high school education, or never smoked. Racial and ethnic disparities were also seen, with non-Hispanic blacks twice as likely to be edentulous as non-Hispanic whites and Mexican Americans[24] (**Table 4**).

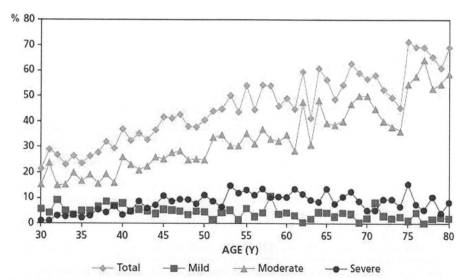

Fig. 2. Prevalence of periodontitis classified by the Centers for Disease Control and Prevention/American Academy of Periodontology case definitions according to age among dentate adults 30 years or older: total (mild, moderate, or severe; *aqua*), mild (*brown*), moderate (*green*), and severe (*blue*) periodontitis; National Health and Nutrition Examination Survey 2009 to 2014 (N = 10,683). (*From* Eke PI, Thornton-Evans GO, Wei L, Borgnakke WS, Dye BA, Genco RJ. Periodontitis in US Adults: National Health and Nutrition Examination Survey 2009-2014. J Am Dent Assoc. 2018 Jul;149(7):576-588.e6. https://doi.org/10.1016/j.adaj.2018.04.023. PMID: 29957185; with permission.)

Table 4
Percentage of adults aged 65 y or older who have lost all their natural teeth, by selected characteristics, United States, National Health and Nutrition Examination Survey, 1999 to 2004 and 2011 to 2016

Characteristic	1999–2004		2011–2016		Change %[a]
	%	SE	%	SE	
Total	27.2	1.44	17.3	1.31	−9.9[b]
Age (y)					
65–74[c]	24.0	1.53	13.0	1.30	−11.0[b]
≥75	31.2	1.83	22.5[b]	1.63	−8.7[b]
Sex					
Male[c]	24.5	1.58	17.7	1.51	−6.8[b]
Female	29.2	1.61	16.9	1.31	−12.3[b]
Race and ethnicity					
White, non-Hispanic[c]	25.9	1.66	15.2	1.66	−10.7[b]
Black, non-Hispanic	33.7	2.47	30.7[b]	2.09	−3.0
Mexican American	24.4	2.56	16.7	1.89	−7.6[b]
Poverty status					
<100% FPL	43.8	3.71	34.1[b]	2.99	−9.7[b]
100% to 199% FPL	36.1	2.14	26.1[b]	2.27	−10.0[b]
≥200% FPL[c]	17.3	1.27	10.7	1.30	−6.6[b]
Poverty status					
<200% FPL	38.4	1.91	28.6[b]	1.95	−9.7[b]
≥200% FPL[c]	17.3	1.27	10.7	1.30	−6.6[b]
Education					
< High school	43.0	2.61	34.8[b]	2.12	−8.2[b]
High school	28.3	2.36	21.3[b]	2.19	−6.9[b]
> High school[c]	13.6	1.09	9.3	1.06	−4.3[b]
Cigarette smoking history					
Current smoker	49.7	3.20	42.8[b]	3.12	−6.9
Former smoker	28.8	1.96	18.5[b]	1.31	−10.2[b]
Never smoked[c]	21.5	1.69	12.1	1.14	−9.4[b]

Note: All estimates are adjusted by age (5-y groups; maximum age group is >80) to the US 2000 standard population.

Abbreviations: SE, standard error; FPL, federal poverty level; less than 100% FPL = poor; 100% to 199% FPL = near poor; less than 200% FPL = poor and near poor combined; and ≥200% FPL = not poor.

[a] Change in percentage points from 1999 to 2004 to 2011 to 2016. Positive value = increase; negative value = decrease.

[b] P <.05 based on *t* test for differences between 2 periods or 2 groups within each characteristic.

[c] Reference group for comparisons within each characteristic, 2011 to 2016.

From Eke PI, Thornton-Evans GO, Wei L, Borgnakke WS, Dye BA, Genco RJ. Periodontitis in US Adults: National Health and Nutrition Examination Survey 2009-2014. J Am Dent Assoc. 2018 Jul;149(7):576-588.e6.   https://doi.org/10.1016/j.adaj.2018.04.023.   PMID: 29957185;   with permission.

During the same timeframe, the mean number of teeth retained by adults aged 65 to 74 years of age was 21.7 (an increase of 2 teeth) and was 19.5 teeth (an increase of 1 tooth) among those aged 75 years or older. Older adults who were non-Hispanic black, Mexican American, or poor, who had less than a high school education, or who were current smokers had no increase in mean number of teeth retained.[24] Again, this suggests an increased need for dental treatment in older adults, regardless of age.

Other measures of tooth loss, retaining all teeth and having a functional dentition (21 or more natural teeth), are also important indicators of oral health status. A positive sign is that the percentage of adults 50 years and older who retained all of their teeth increased from 14% to 21% between 1999 to 2004 and 2009 to 2014. However, these improvements, seen in the general population, were attributable mostly to nonpoor ($\geq$200% federal poverty guideline) older adults.[23] Similarly, a higher percentage of older adults had a functional dentition in 2009 to 2014 than in 1999 to 2004 (67% vs 55%), although the increases generally were significant only for those not living in poverty.[23]

It is important to underscore that the improvements seen in tooth loss measures have been most significant among the nonpoor. Therefore, although overall the aging population is experiencing less edentulism and greater tooth retention, ultimately requiring more preventive and restorative care, poor older adults are at higher risk for tooth loss and should be considered for comprehensive preventive treatment plans aimed at preventing tooth loss.

Oral Cancer

In 2017, it was estimated that 383,415 people in the United States lived with "oral cancer," a term that includes cancers of the oral cavity and oropharynx. The American Cancer Society estimates that 53,260 individuals will be diagnosed with oral cancer in 2020.[18] The rates of oral cancer have risen on average 0.8% each year over the past decade.[18] However, reporting oral cancer rates as a combination of oral cavity and oropharyngeal cancers masks the important fact that cancers of the oral cavity, which have as the major risk factors tobacco use and alcohol consumption, have been declining while oropharyngeal cancer incidence has been increasing.[25] Recently, human papillomavirus (HPV) infection has been recognized as a major risk factor for oropharyngeal cancer and is responsible for a portion of the increase in oropharyngeal cancer in non-Hispanic white men and women. There are differences in outcomes between HPV-positive and HPV-negative oropharyngeal squamous cell cancer, with people having better survival outcomes if HPV-positive.[26] The 5-year relative survival rate for oral cancer is 66.2%. Unfortunately, age-adjusted oral cancer mortalities have risen an average of 0.5% each year, and an estimated 10,750 people in the United States will die from these cancers in 2020.[18] The highest percentage of oral cancer deaths is seen in older adults aged 65 to 74, and median age of death from oral cancer is 68 years.[18]

Oral cancers show marked age and gender disparities. Adults aged 55 to 64 (31.1%) had the highest rates of oral cancer diagnosis.[18] However, individuals aged 50 to 69 had a substantially higher risk for oropharyngeal cancer compared with cancers of the oral cavity. Individuals who were 70 years old or older had higher risk for cancers in the oral cavity as compared with the oropharynx.[25] Despite the fact that the prevalence of oral cancer increases with age, 1 out of 4 cases will occur in patients younger than 55 years old. There are also marked disparities based on gender, with men being afflicted by oral cancer more than 2.5 times as often as women. Historically, black men experienced the highest incidence of oral cancer.[18,27] However, from 2000 to 2010, a break in this trend was documented, and non-Hispanic white men had the highest age-adjusted incidence of oral cancer. During this decade, black men experienced a decrease in both cancer of the oral cavity and cancer of the oropharynx, whereas white men showed an increase in oropharyngeal cancer.[25] Recent data show that this trend continues with rates of new cases of oral cancer per 100,000 persons being 18.1 for white men and 13.3 for black men.[18]

There are also significant and persistent racial disparities in survival rates. The average 5-year survival for blacks has been reported at 48% compared with 67% in whites.[18] A contributing factor to this disparity is that black patients tend to present with more advanced disease than white patients. One study found that 16% of black men and 13% of black women present with metastatic disease, compared with 9% and 8% in white men and women, and that only 17% of African American men are diagnosed with localized disease, compared with 32% of white men.[28] However, even when controlling for stage of diagnosis, blacks have a lower 5-year survival rate than all other racial and ethnic groups, and this racial disparity is seen consistently across age groups.[18]

Social determinants of health have been assessed in those diagnosed with oral cancer in an attempt to understand the cause of this racial disparity. Research has shown that African American patients with oral cancer lived in census block groups with lower education levels, income, and a higher percentage of the population below the poverty line compared with white patients.[29,30] Poorer survival in African Americans was also associated with the traditional risk factors associated with poor oral cancer outcomes, such as alcohol abuse. The analysis also showed racial disparity by insurance status. After controlling for socioeconomic factors, including insurance status, the racial disparities in oral cancer outcomes were greatly diminished, although not eliminated.[28]

In summary, there has been a shift in the epidemiology of oral cancer. For more than a decade, the overall rate of oral cancer has increased slightly each year, but this information is not as clinically useful as if the disease patterns of the 2 distinct groups of cancers that comprise oral cancer are looked at. Cancer of the oral cavity is declining, but older men, especially black men, are at higher risk than older women.[31] The primary risk factors for cancers of the oral cavity are tobacco and alcohol use. Conversely, cancers of the oropharynx are increasing, largely driven by the increase in HPV-positive—related oropharyngeal cancers that are more often found in young, white men. These shifts have implications for changes in clinical practice, including new risk assessment protocols, patient education, and medical/dental collaborations revolving around HPV vaccinations as a way to eliminate the increase in HPV-related oral cancers.

Long-Term Care

In 2016, the estimated number of older adults in the United States was 49.2 million,[32] but only about 3% (1.5 million) lived in long-term care facilities, 1.1 million of those in nursing homes. There was significant disparities by age. Only 16% of nursing home residents were younger than 65. The rate increased only slightly, to 18.2%, for those aged 65 to 74. However, a significant increase was seen for those aged 75 to 84 (26.7%) and those older than 85 years old (38.6%).[33] Still, this is only 9% of persons aged 85 and over,[32] meaning that most of even the oldest old are community dwelling. The projected growth of the older adult population will likely lead to a significant increase in the number of long-term care residents. There are no national data regarding the oral health of older adults in long-term care settings. NHANES data include only community-dwelling older adults, and there is no similar survey for long-term care residents. Consequently, the current oral health status data are gathered from smaller studies. Unfortunately, these studies have shown that the oral health of long-term care residents has been poor.[34,35]

This poor oral health status occurs despite federal regulations that are designed to facilitate good oral health in this vulnerable population. Nursing home facilities are required to provide assistance with activities of daily living, including basic oral hygiene care. In addition, all residents must have a comprehensive assessment that includes an evaluation of their dental status. However, the dental assessment can be done by nursing staff even though all facilities are required to contract with dental personnel.[36] Unfortunately, there are no specific requirements in the regulations regarding the scope of dental services provided as part of the contract, and having a signed contract does not guarantee that needed dental services are provided to the residents. It is important to note that states can expand the regulations on nursing facilities, so reviewing state-specific regulations before entering into an agreement with a nursing home is prudent.

Unfortunately, there are few regulations that improve access to dental treatment of nursing home residents. Just as with community-dwelling older adults, Medicare does not cover dental services. The daily nursing facility fee paid by Medicare does not cover a resident's dental care outside of daily hygiene. Dental treatment, including examinations and preventive services, is the financial responsibility of the resident or their family, irrespective of whether the care is provided onsite at the nursing home or at a community dental office. Facilities are required to assist residents with Medicaid in obtaining dental care that is covered under the state's Medicaid benefits.[36] Because adult Medicaid benefits vary by state and Medicare Expansion plans often do have comprehensive dental benefits, many nursing home residents or their families need to cover the costs of dental treatment.

Even if finances were not a barrier, although some facilities may provide dental services on site, in most cases the residents must be transported to a dental office in the community. Given that the residents often have chronic diseases, functional impairments, and cognitive decline, it can be challenging to transport the residents for care and difficult-to-find dental providers who are both willing to and feel competent to treat the residents.[37] With all of these challenges, one can readily understand why reports of poor oral health in long-term care facilities are common. The residents' complex medical and functional conditions both increase their risk for oral disease and decrease their ability to easily access the care they need.

One multisite study that documented residents' oral health status was conducted in 1226 nursing home residents in 23 nursing homes without onsite dental services. The purpose of the study was to evaluate the residents' oral health status and assess the impact of age, gender, care dependency, and income level on their oral health status and treatment needs. The residents' mean age was 83.9 years, and 41.9% were edentulous. More than 3 out of 4 (77%) of residents needed extractions or fillings. Of the residents wearing removable dentures, 36.9% of the dentures needed repair, rebasing, or replacement. The mixed model analysis showed that with each year a resident ages, the oral health outcomes get worse and that men have worse oral health and higher treatment needs than women. However, income and care dependency had little effect in predicting the oral health outcomes. This finding could be due to the relative homogeneity of these factors in long-term care settings. In summary, the nursing home residents presented a poor overall oral health status and higher dental and prosthetic treatment needs than the general population of older adults in the United States.[38]

This study confirms the findings of previous studies, which found long-term care residents have substantially poorer oral health than the general US population. In order to address this disparity, many factors will need to be addressed, including improving access to high-quality dental care for long-term care residents, expanding financing of dental care for older adults, enhancing the predoctoral and postdoctoral dental education curriculum, so dentists are better prepared to provide care for this challenging population, and creating policies that require higher levels/standards of oral health care in long-term care facilities.

SUMMARY

The projected shift in the demographics of US older adults predicts a larger and more diverse group who retains their teeth longer than previous generations. Because there are significant oral health disparities related to race, ethnicity, gender, and income, these demographic trends are likely to translate into a dramatic increase in oral disease, a corresponding increase in treatment needs, and increased demand for services. In order to eliminate oral health disparities in older adults, the dental profession must advocate for health policies that promote tooth retention and the maintenance of good oral health in all populations of older adults. For example, the inclusion of a comprehensive dental benefit in Medicare has the potential to significantly reduce oral health disparities by ensuring equitable access to dental care. On an individual practitioner level, dentists must develop and ensure access to culturally appropriate clinical care. Because culturally sensitive care has been shown to improve health outcomes,[39] new accreditation standards for dental and dental hygiene schools require that dental graduates are competent in providing culturally appropriate care. In addition, many organizations offer continuing education courses that provide cultural competence and sensitivity training. Dental professionals will need these skills in order to be effective members of an interdisciplinary team that appropriately tailors care to older adults, based not only on disease risk but also on cultural beliefs, comorbid conditions, frailty, cognitive function, and physical function. When successful, and oral health status is improved, this has the potential to positively affect overall health, prevent physical decline, and improve quality of life.[40]

CLINICS CARE POINTS

- Most oral diseases are preventable, but older adults experience oral health disparities.
- Good oral health is vital to general health and quality of life, yet older adults are at increased risk for oral diseases, especially older adults with lower incomes and from minority racial and ethnic groups.
- As the population of older adults becomes more racially and ethnically diverse, the demographics of dental patients will reflect those changes.
- Providing culturally sensitive care will be necessary in order to ensure optimal, patient-centered care for the increasingly diverse population of older adults.
- Given older adults' increased risk for caries and periodontal disease, new clinical approaches and preventive strategies will be needed for effective management.

REFERENCES

1. Gil-Montoya JA, de Mello AL, Barrios R, et al. Oral health in the elderly patient and its impact on general well-being: a nonsystematic review. Clin Interv Aging 2015; 10:461–7.
2. U.S. Department of Health and Human Services. Oral Health in America: A Report of the Surgeon General. Rockville (MD): U.S. Department of Health and Human Services, National Institute of Dental and Craniofacial Research, National Institutes of Health; 2000.
3. U.S. Department of Health and Human Services, Office of Disease Prevention and Health Promotion. Healthy people. Washington, DC: U.S. Department of

Health and Human Services, Office of Disease Prevention and Health Promotion; 2020. Available at: https://www.healthypeople.gov/2020/about/foundation-health-measures/Disparities. Accessed November 8, 2020.

4. Whitehead M. The concepts and principles of equity and health. Int J Health Serv 1992;22(3):429–45.
5. Braveman P. What are health disparities and health equity? We need to be clear. Public Health Rep 2014;129(Suppl 2):5–8.
6. Braveman P. Health difference, disparity, inequality or inequity–what difference does it make what we call it?. In: Buchbinder M, Rivkin-Fish M, Walker RL, editors. Understanding health inequalities and justice. Chapel Hill (NC): The University of North Carolina Press; 2016. p. 33–63.
7. Association APH. Social justice and health 2020. Available at: https://apha.org/what-is-public-health/generation-public-health/our-work/social-justice. Accessed November 17, 2020.
8. Maguire A. Illustrating equality vs equity. In: Interaction Institute for Social Change; 2016.
9. Organization WH. Social determinants of health 2020. Available at: https://www.who.int/health-topics/social-determinants-of-health#tab=tab_1. Accessed November 17, 2020.
10. Ending racial and ethnic health disparities in the USA. Lancet 2011;377(9775): 1379.
11. Fisher-Owens SA, Gansky SA, Platt LJ, et al. Influences on children's oral health: a conceptual model. Pediatrics 2007;120(3):e510–20.
12. Henshaw MM, Garcia RI, Weintraub JA. Oral health disparities across the life span. Dent Clin North Am 2018;62(2):177–93.
13. Issrani R, Ammanagi R, Keluskar V. Geriatric dentistry–meet the need. Gerodontology 2012;29(2):e1–5.
14. Griffin SO, Jones JA, Brunson D, et al. Burden of oral disease among older adults and implications for public health priorities. Am J Public Health 2012;102(3): 411–8.
15. Kelley J, Han C, Iqbal A, et al. Oral health disparities among older adults: race/ethnicity, lifestyle, and structural access to care. Innov Aging 2018; 2(suppl_1):648.
16. Wu B, Liang J, Plassman BL, et al. Oral health among white, black, and Mexican-American elders: an examination of edentulism and dental caries. J Public Health Dent 2011;71(4):308–17.
17. National Health and Nutrition Examination Survey [Internet]. CDC/National Center for Health Statistics. CDC/National Center for Health Statistics. Available at: https://www.cdc.gov/nchs/nhanes/index.htm. Accessed July 27, 2017.
18. National Cancer Institute S. Epidemiology, and End Results Program. Cancer Stat Facts: oral cavity and pharynx cancer. Available at: https://seer.cancer.gov/statfacts/html/oralcav.html. Accessed November 17, 2020.
19. Prevention CfDCa. Dental Caries Among Adults and Older Adults. Centers for Disease Control and Prevention, US Dept of Health and Human Services. Oral Health Surveillance Report: trends in dental caries and sealants, tooth retention, and edentulism, United States, 1999–2004 to 2011–2016. Web site. 2019. Available at: https://www.cdc.gov/oralhealth/publications/OHSR-2019-dental-carries-adults.html. Accessed November 8, 2020.
20. Eke PI, Thornton-Evans GO, Wei L, et al. Periodontitis in US adults: National Health and Nutrition Examination Survey 2009-2014. J Am Dent Assoc 2018; 149(7):576–88.e6.

21. Eke PI, Wei L, Thornton-Evans GO, et al. Risk indicators for periodontitis in US adults: NHANES 2009 to 2012. J Periodontol 2016;87(10):1174–85.
22. Eke PI, Dye BA, Wei L, et al. CDC Periodontal Disease Surveillance Workgroup: James Beck GDRP. Prevalence of periodontitis in adults in the United States: 2009 and 2010. J Dent Res 2012;91(10):914–20.
23. Dye BA, Weatherspoon DJ, Lopez Mitnik G. Tooth loss among older adults according to poverty status in the United States from 1999 through 2004 and 2009 through 2014. J Am Dent Assoc 2019;150(1):9–23.e3.
24. Prevention CfDCa. Edentulism and tooth retention. Centers for Disease Control and Prevention, US Dept of Health and Human Services. Oral Health Surveillance report: trends in dental caries and sealants, tooth retention, and edentulism, United States, 1999–2004 to 2011–2016. Web site. 2019. Available at: https://www.cdc.gov/oralhealth/publications/OHSR-2019-edentulism-tooth-retention.html#Aged65. Accessed November 8, 2020.
25. Weatherspoon DJ, Chattopadhyay A, Boroumand S, et al. Oral cavity and oropharyngeal cancer incidence trends and disparities in the United States: 2000-2010. Cancer Epidemiol 2015;39(4):497–504.
26. Dalianis T. Human papillomavirus and oropharyngeal cancer, the epidemics, and significance of additional clinical biomarkers for prediction of response to therapy (review). Int J Oncol 2014;44(6):1799–805.
27. Morse DE, Kerr AR. Disparities in oral and pharyngeal cancer incidence, mortality and survival among black and white Americans. J Am Dent Assoc 2006;137(2):203–12.
28. Goodwin WJ, Thomas GR, Parker DF, et al. Unequal burden of head and neck cancer in the United States. Head Neck 2008;30(3):358–71.
29. Molina MA, Cheung MC, Perez EA, et al. African American and poor patients have a dramatically worse prognosis for head and neck cancer: an examination of 20,915 patients. Cancer 2008;113(10):2797–806.
30. Gourin CG, Podolsky RH. Racial disparities in patients with head and neck squamous cell carcinoma. Laryngoscope 2006;116(7):1093–106.
31. LeHew CW, Weatherspoon DJ, Peterson CE, et al. The health system and policy implications of changing epidemiology for oral cavity and oropharyngeal cancers in the United States from 1995 to 2016. Epidemiol Rev 2017;39(1):132–47.
32. Roberts AW, Ogunwole SU, Blakeslee L, et al. The population 65 years and older in the United States: 2016. Washington, DC: U.S. Census Bureau; 2018.
33. Harris-Kojetin LSM, Lendon JP, Rome V, et al. Long-term care providers and services users in the United States, 2015–2016. Hyattsville (MD): National Center for Health Statistics; 2019.
34. Ziebolz D, Werner C, Schmalz G, et al. Oral health and nutritional status in nursing home residents-results of an explorative cross-sectional pilot study. BMC Geriatr 2017;17(1):39.
35. Chen X, Clark JJ, Naorungroj S. Oral health in nursing home residents with different cognitive statuses. Gerodontology 2013;30(1):49–60.
36. Dental services. In: Health and Human Services, 42 § 483.55: C.F.R., 1991.
37. Hoben M, Clarke A, Huynh KT, et al. Barriers and facilitators in providing oral care to nursing home residents, from the perspective of care aides: a systematic review and meta-analysis. Int J Nurs Stud 2017;73:34–51.
38. Janssens B, Vanobbergen J, Petrovic M, et al. The oral health condition and treatment needs assessment of nursing home residents in Flanders (Belgium). Community Dent Health 2017;34(3):143–51.

39. Tucker CM, Marsiske M, Rice KG, et al. Patient-centered culturally sensitive health care: model testing and refinement. Health Psychol 2011;30(3):342–50.
40. Tonetti MS, Bottenberg P, Conrads G, et al. Dental caries and periodontal diseases in the ageing population: call to action to protect and enhance oral health and well-being as an essential component of healthy ageing - consensus report of group 4 of the joint EFP/ORCA workshop on the boundaries between caries and periodontal diseases. J Clin Periodontol 2017;44(Suppl 18):S135–44.

Physiology of Aging of Older Adults

Systemic and Oral Health Considerations— 2021 Update

Lisa A. Thompson, DMD[a], Helen Chen, MD[b,c],*

KEYWORDS

• Physiology • Aging adults • Oral health • Normal aging • Age-dependent changes
• Systemic • Clinical significance

KEY POINTS

- There is greater physiologic heterogeneity in older adults than in younger cohorts, which makes clinical care more complex for the geriatric practitioner.
- Normal physiologic changes associated with aging different from the disease process and warrant an in-depth understanding and application for patient-centered care.
- Cardiovascular and pulmonary changes associated with normal aging can result in vital sign lability, reduced tolerance for prolonged procedures, and need for special considerations regarding patient positioning.
- Metabolic changes related to liver or kidney function may require alternate drug selection or dose adjustments of commonly used medications, such as antibiotics.
- Older adults may have multiple physiologic changes that combine, leading to increased risk for frailty and poorer oral health.

INTRODUCTION

As 2030 approaches, the decade all baby boomers will be over the age of 65, providers must be prepared to provide up-to-date comprehensive care for aging patients. As the population ages, it becomes more heterogeneous, with a wider distribution of physiologic reserve for each individual. Cognitive status, chronic multiple diseases, and medications add to the physiologic heterogeneity of this population. In simple terms, healthy older adults are more unlike each other than are equally healthy

This article has been updated from a version previously published in Dental Clinics of North America, Volume 58, Issue 4, October 2014.

[a] Geriatric Dental Fellowship, Harvard School of Dental Medicine, 188 Longwood Avenue, Boston, MA 02115, USA; [b] Hebrew SeniorLife, Boston, MA, USA; [c] Division of Gerontology, Beth Israel Deaconess Medical Center, Harvard Medical School, Boston, MA, USA
* Corresponding author. Hebrew Rehabilitation Center, 1200 Centre Street, Roslindale, MA 02131.
E-mail address: helenchen@hsl.harvard.edu

younger adults in most studies of physiologic function. Although less thoroughly studied, oral health changes over the life span appear to observe the same principles of normative physiologic aging as other organ systems and physiologic processes. Oral aging is as relevant as any other health care challenge facing an aging society. Many well-studied physiologic functions of the older adult population have an impact on the oral cavity. Many of these physiologic changes contribute to the lower threshold for developing oral disease, nutritional and swallowing problems, taste and smell impairment, chronic pain, and psychological distress. As information and research on normative changes with aging have emerged, this material has been updated to confirm and reinforce what already is known with new information on normal aging and the clinical significance of normal aging of older adults. This article reviews the concepts of physiologic reserve; normative aging processes of the cardiovascular, metabolic, and musculoskeletal systems that are applicable to oral health; and age-related changes in the oral cavity and the clinical significance of those changes. This article is not meant to focus on diseases related to aging but rather to begin to explore the normal physiologic changes associated with aging dentition and systemic changes with age for a better understanding of the presentation of older adults and how it may change the approach to diagnosis and treatment.

PHYSIOLOGY OF AGING

First, when considering aging physiology, it is important to understand that the line between normative aging and disease is uncertain. Despite this, aging alone changes the physiologic threshold at which individuals can withstand physiologic challenges due to stressful occurrences, such as surgery, illness, injury, and severe environmental conditions. In older adults, physiologic reserve is reduced and the ability to maintain healthy physiologic balance is blunted. For example, an older adult given an intravenous salt load may lack the cardiac or renal reserve to adapt to sodium and volume shifts. Studies reveal that healthy older adults have stiffer hearts and, therefore, do not get as much ventricular stretch and Starling curve–induced increased cardiac output with this volume expansion. Changes in the autonomic nervous system also may lead to a loss of variation in heart rate response to stimuli. Even in the healthy older adult, the ability to increase heart rate is limited and impedes the cardiorenal system from filtering salt as rapidly or efficiently as younger adults. This lowered threshold for maintaining homeostasis, coined *homeostenosis*, results from a decreased ability of physiologic systems to modulate such deviations from physiologic baselines. In describing systemic physiologic changes, it becomes hard to isolate each system because of the interconnectedness needed to adapt and maintain normal functioning. Multiple systemic physiologic changes also can combine to contribute to frailty and functional decline. The next section more specifically explores the relationship between known normative age-related changes in physiology and their impact on oral health.

Systemic Changes Associated with Oral Health

Cardiovascular
Normal cardiovascular changes with age are both structural and functional. There is an overall decreased cardiovascular reserve with a loss of and hypertrophy of myocytes; 90% of pacemaker cells in the sinus node are lost by the age of 75,[1] resulting in slower resting and maximum heart rates. As described by Cefalu and colleagues,[1] normal aging increases stiffness of the left ventricle, resulting in a decrease in left ventricular compliance. Even with the addition of left ventricular filling that results with

atrial contraction, the normal aged left ventricle creates a higher left ventricular end-diastolic pressure, a more robust Starling curve position point, and a higher stroke volume as the ventricle moves from diastole to systole. Arterial stiffness, the result of age-related calcification and collagen deposition in place of elastin, coupled with decreased nitrous oxide vasodilator effects, raises systolic vascular resistance, further impeding forward flow, increasing myocardial oxygen demand and cardiac work. In addition to the aforementioned normative changes in left ventricular function, the aging heart experiences decreasing abilities to raise heart rate and has more muted responses to cholinergic and sympathomimetic stimulation. This limits the heart's ability to respond to additional stress. This results in an increased risk of congestive heart failure in the presence of chronic disease processes, such as diabetes, hypertension, and coronary heart disease.[1] Despite these changes, the cardiovascular system compensates to maintain function but may have difficulty adapting under stressors, such as a dental appointment.[2]

In the dental office, it is important to understand blood pressure changes found in older adults. With the normal aging heart, blood pressure tends to increase partially due to increased aortic and arterial stiffness. Systolic pressure has been known to rise continuously with age whereas diastolic pressure fluctuates with age, leading to an increase in pulse pressure. In adults over the age of 50, increased pulse pressure and systolic blood pressure greater than 140 mm Hg are more significant risk factors for heart disease than diastolic blood pressure.[3,4] Hypertension, a risk factor for cardiovascular disease and one of the most common medical conditions among adults older than 75, affects approximately two-thirds and three-fourths of men and women, respectively.[5] Older adults with systolic blood pressure greater than 150 mm Hg merit referral for initiation or intensification of treatment.[6] Additionally, because of blunted baroreceptors in the carotid arteries that do not modulate acute changes in blood pressure in normal aging, oral health providers also must be aware of postural hypotension likely to occur in normal individuals on standing from a sitting or lying position in the dental chair.[1]

Pulmonary

Normal structural changes with age in the respiratory system include stiffening of the rib cage and alterations in connective tissue with reduced diaphragmatic and intercostal muscle strength, including early fatigue of the diaphragm, decreased perception of dyspnea, and reduced airway size and shallower alveolar cells and sacs, which result in decreased vital capacity and forced expiratory volume with an increase in residual volume and functional residual capacity.[1] Although all these changes are considered normal, these physiologic changes lower the threshold for adaptive ability, increase the risk of disease, and have an effect on oral health.

Many of these changes contribute to a decreased cough reflex and defective mucus clearance directly impacting oral health through an increase the risk of aspiration both in the dental chair during treatment and of plaque accumulation on teeth and dentures.[7] Additionally, normative changes with age associated with decreased genioglossal reflex and an elongated soft palate increase the risk for obstructive sleep apnea and hypertension secondary to obstructive sleep apnea.

Liver

As the liver ages, it decreases in size by approximately 1% every year beginning at age 40 and, as the aging process continues, blood flow to the liver decreases by 40% to 45%.[8] In vivo and in vitro studies also have shown a decrease in hepatic metabolic activity, further reducing liver function with age.[9] These changes affect hepatic drug metabolism and clearance and should be taken into consideration when prescribing medications.

Kidney

The normal aging kidney undergoes structural and physiologic changes that may compromise function, such as decreases in renal blood flow, glomerular and tubular mass, and glomerular filtration rate (GFR). By age 40, the GFR declines by a rate of 1% per year. Despite this, fluid homeostasis generally is maintained. For older adults with and without chronic kidney disease, renal excretion of medications takes longer than younger adults.[1,8,10]

The clinical importance in dentistry of renal physiologic changes due to aging are related primarily to prescribing. Classes of drugs commonly prescribed by dentists in which renal dose adjustment is important to prevent side effects include fluroquinolones (phototoxicity, hallucinations, delusions, seizures, and cognitive dysfunction), penicillins (seizures and cognitive dysfunction), fluconazole, and aminoglycoside antibiotics.[1,11] Additionally, some opioids, such as morphine and hydromorphone, have metabolites that are excreted in the kidneys and should be used with increased caution in older adults.

Musculoskeletal

In the normal aging process of the musculoskeletal system, there is a decline in bone mineralization and architectural strength of the bony matrices; microfractures accumulate and joints stiffen as a result of a decline in water content in the tendons, ligaments, cartilage, and synovial compartments.[1] Additionally, both muscle mass and total body water decrease with an increase in total body fat. This decreases the volume of distribution of water-soluble medications, such as penicillin, effectively concentrating the dose in older adults compared with younger adults. Conversely, the distribution of lipid-soluble medications increases and drugs, such as diazepam and lidocaine, may reach lower serum concentrations but have a longer half-life due to distribution throughout adipose tissue.[8]

Normal age-related functional changes also may include a greater loss of strength in the lower extremities compared with the upper extremities but with a reduction in hand grip strength.[1] In healthy but frailer individuals, this could affect tooth brushing and flossing ability and efficiency. Adaptive devices and tooth brush modifications may need to be made to accommodate an individual's ability. Gait speed and the ability to change position or tolerate positioning also may be impacted by normal musculoskeletal changes with aging, which may require modifications in the physical layout of the dental office and considerations in scheduling.

In summary, due to diminished physiologic reserve of the cardiopulmonary, metabolic, and musculoskeletal systems associated with the aging process and possible comorbidities, the body's ability to respond to external stress decreases. To decrease potential external stress, it is important to take into consideration appointment time, duration, and procedure type when scheduling older adult patients and prescribing for them.

Frailty and oral health

Frailty as a geriatric syndrome is characterized by the presence of weight loss, fatigue, weakness, and decreased physical activity.[12] Although not considered part of normal aging, frailty is more prevalent as older adults age and increases the risk for disablement, hospitalization, and mortality. The risk for developing frailty is increased by the presence of functional decline and multiple comorbidities, and frailty can increase the risk for further functional decline. For example, an older adult with decreased cardiopulmonary and musculoskeletal reserve may become easily fatigued during meals, and basic hygiene tasks, contributing to weight loss, poorer oral hygiene, and a negative feedback loop that contributes to increased frailty.

In summary, due to diminished physiologic reserve of the cardiopulmonary, metabolic, and musculoskeletal systems associated with the aging process and possible comorbidities, the body's ability to respond to external stress decreases. To decrease potential external stress, it is important to take into consideration appointment time, duration, and procedure type when scheduling older adult patients and prescribing for them.

Oral/Pharyngeal Changes

The normal aging process of the oral cavity undergoes many physiologic changes; however, many of these changes are secondary due to chronic systemic disease and their treatment regiments (inflammatory response, medication, chemotherapy, and radiotherapy).[13] This section focuses on the normative changes in the aging oral cavity and the clinical significance of those changes rather than pathologic changes associated with disease, trauma, and unnatural wear.

Dentition

Due to a variety of factors, older adults are retaining more of their natural teeth; however, tooth retention varies widely with socioeconomic status.[14] Aging changes in tooth anatomy and histology depend on chemical and mechanical wear from mastication as well as factors, such as culture, diet, occupation, tooth composition, and resiliency and strength of teeth and the surrounding periodontal apparatus.[15] There has not been a significant amount of research documenting changes in the dentition since the last publication; the clinical significance to normative age-related changes for the dental practitioner is highlighted.

Enamel Enamel is composed of the highest percent of mineral content, making it the hardest tissue in the body.[16] It has been observed that changes occur in both physical appearance and molecular composition in health aging adults, related mainly to the exchange of minerals in the oral environment with the enamel surface and mechanical wear over time.[17]

The demineralization-remineralization process that occurs throughout life has an impact on the enamel hardness and subsequent tooth wear. Additional site-specific wear patterns and changes in enamel thickness have been observed in older adults compared with younger cohorts.[18,19] **Fig. 1** illustrates the thickening and shortening of the enamel at the incisal edge of the tooth and the thinning of the enamel at the cervical third of the tooth at the cement-enamel junction. Signs of overall tooth wear are flattening, darkening, and smoother surfaces due to the loss of the outer enamel surface.

The deeper layers of enamel that are exposed from the chemical-mechanical wear that occurs over time from a tooth's exposure to demineralization-remineralization process and mastication have different physical and chemical properties.[17] A study in 2008 found the elastic modulus and hardness of the outer enamel surface to increase by 16% and 12%, respectively, in old enamel compared with young enamel.[16] Park and colleagues[16] speculate that decreased permeability, increased brittleness, and tooth fracture are caused by an association between the increase in elastic modulus and hardness and the interprismatic organic matrix.

Another age-related change to enamel is the loss of fluoride from the enamel surface[17] and an increase in the fluoride concentration in the cervical third of the tooth.

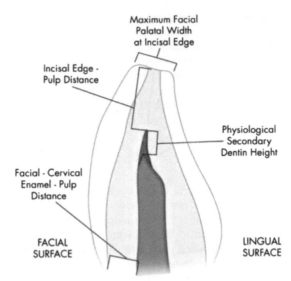

Maximum Facial
Palatal Width
at Incisal Edge

Incisal Edge -
Pulp Distance

Physiological
Secondary
Dentin Height

Facial - Cervical
Enamel - Pulp
Distance

FACIAL
SURFACE

LINGUAL
SURFACE

Fig. 1. Increases with age of physiologic secondary dentin height and incisal edge enamel-pulp distance. (*Courtesy of* Gregory An, DDS, MPH.)

Unfortunately, this is not necessarily protective for caries that develop in the cervical third of the tooth that initially develop on the root dentin surfaces.

The clinical significance of these changes to the enamel is decreased enamel thickness for tooth preparation, decreased hydration, more effective acid etching, smoother and more translucent facial contours, flattened incisal and interproximal wear, cracks along enamel surfaces, and brittleness.[15,17,18]

Dentin Age-related changes in dentin, the mineral, organic, and water-rich layer just below enamel are primarily due to chemical and mechanical impacts related to the formation of secondary dentin as well as sclerosis of the dentinal tubules. The pulp chamber occurs primarily in the mesial-distal direction and then in the vestibular-oral direction at approximately 60 years to 70 years old.[17,20,21] These changes contribute to a reduction in tubular fluid movement and subsequent deceased dentinal hypersensitivity. Additional age-related changes lead to higher calcium concentration in dentin as well as higher hardness and elastic modulus.[22] Although not conclusive, 1 study suggests that age-related decreased strength of root dentin and fracture toughness may contribute to a higher rate of spontaneous vertical root fracture in older adults.[22]

The clinical significance of these changes in increased volume, secondary and reparative dentin, and decreased solubility are change in tooth color, decreased hypersensitivity, and decreased bond strength; to improve retention, use macromechanical strategies in addition to micromechanical and chemical strategies.[23]

Pulp Age-related changes to the pulp decrease the reparative capabilities due to reduction in pulpal blood flow and blood vessels and increased tissue calcification. Older patients have fewer nerve branches, greater mineralization of the dental pulp nerves, and increased connective tissue within the pulp.[24–27] Clinical significance of these changes lead to delay responses to thermal stimuli and decreased sensitivity and pain perception. Thermal pulp testing may be ineffective or result in increased false-negative responses[17] depending on calcification of the pulp space. Electric pulp testing may be required.[28,29]

Cementum Cementum is a mineralized tissue that encases the tooth root attaching the tooth to the periodontium mediated through the cementum-dentin junction. Normative age-related changes occur most significantly at the apical third of the root (**Fig. 2**), which bears the greatest occlusal load during mastication[30] as well as a gross increase in cementum hardness.[30] An increased exposure of cementum from gingival recession may result in hypercementosis. The clinical significance of these age-related changes is decreased sensitivity to thermal stimuli and reporting of pain.[15]

Figs. 1 and **2** illustrate some of the anatomic changes that take place within enamel, dentin, pulpal tissue, and cementum.

Periodontal apparatus
The periodontal apparatus is composed of the tissues that attach the tooth to the alveolar process—gingiva, cementum, periodontal ligament, and alveolar bone. Age-related changes alone do not cause clinically significant periodontal attachment apparatus loss—rather, the presence of disease and the inflammatory process in combination to biomolecular changes of the periodontal cells.[31] Epidemiologic studies show a higher prevalence of periodontal disease in older cohorts compared with younger cohorts most likely due to cumulative tissue destruction over a lifetime rather than age-dependent risk of periodontal susceptibility.[28,32,33]

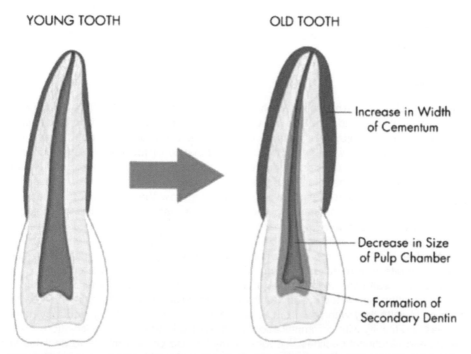

YOUNG TOOTH   OLD TOOTH

Increase in Width of Cementum

Decrease in Size of Pulp Chamber

Formation of Secondary Dentin

Fig. 2. Changes to dentin with aging. The secondary dentin grows inwardly into the pulp chamber, decreasing the chamber's size. (*Courtesy of* Gregory An, DDS, MPH.)

Oral mucosa

The function of the oral mucosa is to provide a host defense, mastication, swallowing, speech, and flavor perception.[13] Age-related changes of oral mucosa show a decrease in the elastic fibers and thickening and disorganization of the collagen bundles in the connective tissue. The mucosa becomes less resilient and, with the reduction in the microvasculature, leads to impaired wound healing[34,35] Additionally, changes in oral epithelium were found to enlarge and flatten with age over 50 years.[36] Although there are some notable age-related changes on a cellular level, few clinically significant changes have been observed or reported with respect to appearance or oral sensation.[36,37]

Saliva

Saliva plays in important role in oral health and function. Although there are inconclusive data regarding age-related changes in salivary gland function and production of saliva, reports have identified changes in salivary composition.[36] Specifically, it has been reported that there is an increase in concentration of IgA and a decrease in total protein concentration in saliva[38,39]

The clinical significance to these age-related changes may be thicker and more ropey saliva. Daily oral hygiene practices may need to be more vigilant.

Microbiological changes of the aging oral cavity

The oral microbiome changes in composition and complexity of species colonization as a normative aging process. In healthy adults in their mid-60s, the biofilm microbiota of the periodontium is predominantly gram-positive aerobes. In the later stages of life, enterobacteria, pseudomonads, staphylococci, actinomycetes, and yeasts are more common in the oropharyngeal region compared with earlier stages in life. Additionally, age-related changes in the oral mucosa, discussed previously, can affect immunity and make the oral cavity more susceptible to opportunistic infections by microorganisms and create the conditions to lower the threshold to different microorganisms for developing disease.[40]

SUMMARY

Oral health plays a vital role in several functions that contribute to life quality, longevity, and functional independence. The oral cavity, when functioning properly, provides and contributes to the enjoyment of taste and smell; the appropriate steps needed for deglutition and swallowing and nutrition; maintenance of facial anatomy; and self-esteem. This article focuses on the normative changes in health relative to oral health in aging adults. The age-related changes discussed are independent of disease or medication use and are essential in understanding how these physiologic changes contribute to a lower threshold for developing disease. A decreased physiologic reserve with normal age-related changes in health coupled with decreased access to care can be more difficult to cope with for an older adult compare with a young adult. Older adults are more different from one another physiologically than are younger adults, which makes geriatric care a greater challenge for the clinician.

Good oral health has an impact on quality of life in myriad ways: social interaction, communication, self-esteem, and healthy nutrition. Older adults who have issues with their oral health may withdraw from social activities, including dining, and may have increased difficulty with communication, thus leading to further social isolation, loneliness, and functional declines.[41] Poor oral health also can contribute to declines in overall physical health. The oral health clinician plays a critical role in supporting the overall health, independence, and quality of life for older adults.

CLINICS CARE POINTS

- To decrease potential external stress, it is important to take into consideration appointment time, duration, and procedure type when scheduling older adult patients and prescribing for them.

- Clinically significant changes to the enamel, dentin, cementum, and pulp can have an impact on the need for oral care management and/or treatment and the ideal treatments for older adults.

- A comprehensive understanding of the impact normative changes with aging combined with a comprehensive geriatric assessment and treatment planning consideration is a solid foundation for caring for the oral health of older adults.

DISCLOSURES

Conflict of interest: the authors have nothing to disclose.

REFERENCES

1. Cefalu C. Theories and mechanisms of aging. Clin Geriatr Med 2011;27:491–506.
2. Bergman SA, Coletti D. Perioperative management of the geriatric patient. part ii: cardiovascular system. Oral Surg Oral Med Oral Pathol Oral Radiol Endod 2006; 102:e7–12.
3. Glick M. The new blood pressure guidelines. J Am Dent Assoc 2004;135:585–6.
4. Pinto E. Blood pressure and ageing. Postgrad Med J 2007;83:109–14.
5. Lipsitz LA. A 91-year-old woman with difficult-to-control hypertension: a clinical review. JAMA 2013;310(12):1274–80.
6. Qaseem A, Wilt TJ, Rich R, et al. Pharmacologic treatment of hypertension in adults aged 60 years or older to higher versus lower blood pressure targets: a clinical practice guideline from the American College of Physicians and the American Academy of Family Physicians. Ann Int Med 2017;166(6):430–7.
7. Bergman SA, Coletti D. Perioperative management of the geriatric patient. part I: respiratory system. Oral Surg Oral Med Oral Pathol Oral Radiol Endod 2006;102:e1–6.
8. Szarejko MJ. Dental considerations for geriatric patients. CME Resource. 2012.
9. Zeeh J, Platt D. The aging liver. Gerotology 2002;48:121–7.
10. Colloca G, Santoro M, Gambassi G. Age-related physiologic changes and perioperative management of elderly patients. Surg Oncol 2010;19:124–30.
11. Mangoni AA, Jackson SHD. Age-related changes in pharmacokinetics and pharmakodynamics: basic principles and practical aplications. Br J Clin Pharmacol 2004;57(1):6–14.
12. Fried LP, Tangen CM, Walston J, et al. Frailty in older adults; evidence for a phenotype. J Gerontol A Biol Sci Med Sci 2001;56(3):M146–56.
13. Ship JA. The influence of aging on oral health and consequences for taste and smell. Physiol Behav 1999;66(2):209–15.
14. Griffin SO, Griffin PM, Li CH, et al. Changes in older adults' oral health and disparities: 1999 to 2004 and 2011 to 2016. J Am Geriatr Soc 2019;67(6):1152–7.
15. An G. Normal aging of teeth. Geriatr Aging 2009;12(10):513–7.
16. Park S, Wang DH, Zhang D, et al. Mechanical properties of human enamel as a function of age and location in the tooth. J Mater Sci Mater Med 2008;19: 2317–24.
17. Carvalho TS, Lussi A. Age-related morphological, histological and functional changes in teeth. J Oral Rehabil 2017;44(4):291–8.

18. Atsu SS, Aka PS, Kucukesmen HC, et al. Age-related changes in tooth enamel as measured by electron microscopy: implications for porcelain laminate veneers. J Prosthet Dent 2005;94:336–41.
19. Kidd EA, Richards A, Thylstrup A, et al. The suscep- tibility of 'young' and 'old' human enamel to artificial caries in vitro. Caries Res 1984;18:226–30.
20. Schroeder HE. Age-related changes in the pulp chamber and its wall in human canine teeth. Schweiz Monatsschr Zahnmed 1993;103:141–9.
21. Schroeder HE, Krey G, Preisig E. Age-related changes of the pulpal dentin wall in human front teeth. Schweiz Monatsschr Zahnmed 1990;100:1450–61.
22. Xu H, Zheng Q, Shao Y, et al. The effects of ageing on the biomechanical prop- erties of root dentine and fracture. J Dent 2014;42:305–11.
23. Lopes GC, Vieira LC, Araujo E, et al. Effect of dentin age and acid etching time on den- tin bonding. J Adhes Dent 2011;13:139–45.
24. Jespersen JJ, Hellstein J, Williamson A, et al. Evaluation of dental pulp sensibility tests in a clinical set- ting. J Endod 2014;40:351–4.
25. Jafarzadeh H, Abbott PV. Review of pulp sensibility tests. Part I: general informa- tion and thermal tests. Int Endod J 2010;43:738–62.
26. Farac RV, Morgental RD, Lima RK, et al. Pulp sensibility test in elderly patients. Gerodontology 2012;29:135–9.
27. Johnstone M, Parashos P. Endodontics and the aging patient. Aust Dental J 2015; 60(1 Suppl):20–7.
28. Goodis HE, Rossall JC, Kahn AJ. Endodontic status in older U.S. adults. J Am Dent Assoc 2001;132:1525–30.
29. Ehrmann EH. Pulp testers and pulp testing with particular reference to the use of dry ice. Aust Dent J 1977;22:272–9.
30. Jang A, Lin JD, Choi RM, et al. Adaptive properties of human cementum and cementum dentin junction with age. J Mech Behav Biomed Mater 2014;39:184–96.
31. Huttner EA, Machado DC, Belle de Oliveira R, et al. Effects of human aging on periodontal tissues. Spec Care Dentist 2009;29(4):149–55.
32. Kress B, Buhl Y, Hahnel S, et al. Age- and tooth-related pulp Cavity Signal Changes in Healthy Teeth: a comparative magnetic resonace imaging analysis. Oral Surg Oral Med Oral Pathol Oral Radiol Endod 2007;103(1):134–7.
33. Boehm TK, Scannapieco FA. The epidemiology, consequences and manage- ment of periodontal disease in older adults. J Am Dent Assoc 2007;138(9 supplement):26S–33S.
34. Holm-Pedersen P, Loe H. Wound healing in the gingiva of young and old individ- uals. Scand J Dent Res 1971;79:40–53.
35. Klein DR. Oral soft tissue changes in geriatric patients. Bull N Y Acad Med 1980; 56:721–7.
36. Lamster IB, Asadourian L, Del Carmen T, et al. The aging mouth: differentiating normal aging from disease. Periodontol 2000 2016;72(1):96–107.
37. Calhoun KH, Gibson B, Hartley L, et al. Age-related changes in oral sensation. Laryngoscope 1992;102:109–16.
38. Eliasson L, Birkhed D, Osterberg T, et al. Minor salivary gland secretion rates and immunoglobulin A in adults and the elderly. Eur J Oral Sci 2006;114:494–9.
39. Vissink A, Spijkervet FK, Van Nieuw Amerongen A. Aging, saliva: a review of the literature. Spec Care Dentist 1996;16:95–103.
40. Belibasakis GN. Microbiological changes of the ageing oral cavity. Arch Oral Biol 2018;96:230–2.
41. Rouxel P, Heilmann A, Demakakos P, et al. Oral health related quality of life and loneliness among older adults. Eur J Ageing 2017;14(2):101–9.

Geriatric Phenotypes and Their Impact on Oral Health

Roseann Mulligan, DDS, MS[a],*, Piedad Suarez Durall, DDS, MS[b]

KEYWORDS

- Geriatric dentistry • Multimorbidity • Phenotypes • Edentulism
- Salivary hypofunction • Polypharmacy • Infection and inflammation • Malnutrition

KEY POINTS

- Older adults have multiple morbidities that can complicate their systemic health and their oral health.
- Examining the most common geriatric phenotypes and their relationship to oral disorders helps the practitioner to prepare for and deliver appropriate care.
- Patient-centered dental clinical practice guidelines for older adults are lacking.
- Using the existing guidelines for older adults may lead to fragmented and inefficient care, as well as increased costs.
- Interprofessional teams are important in the dental care of older adults.

INTRODUCTION

Many countries have been tracking the changing proportion of adults 60 years of age and older within their borders, with most demonstrating some level of growth. From a global perspective, individuals 60 years of age and older made up 11% (605 million) of all people; there are projections of the world's population of adults 60 and older doubling to 22% (2 billion) by 2050.[1]

With increasing longevity have come higher rates of morbidity owing to chronic disease. Current studies demonstrate 80% of older adults having at least 1 chronic condition with 40% having 2 or more.[2] This coexistence of chronic systemic diseases has been termed multimorbidity or comorbidity.[3] Epidemiologic studies have shown that multimorbidity is associated with an increased risk of death, disability, poor functional status, poor quality of life, adverse drug events, and other unfavorable results.[4]

Morbidity clusters have also been described, with certain diseases seeming to show a propensity to occur simultaneously, for example, hypertension and diabetes.[5]

This article originally appeared in Dental Clinics, Volume 65 Issue 2, April 2021.
[a] Herman Ostrow School of Dentistry of the University of Southern California, DEN 4338, Mail Code: 0641, Los Angeles, CA 90089, USA; [b] Herman Ostrow School of Dentistry of the University of Southern California, University Park Campus, DEN 4338, Mail Code: 0641, Los Angeles, CA 90089, USA
* Corresponding author.
E-mail address: mulligan@usc.edu

Similarly, comorbidity and clustering can happen with oral conditions, for example, salivary hypofunction and caries. If one were to look at comorbidities across the spectrum of oral, systemic, and psychosocial factors, it is likely that other clusters would be found, potentially influencing each other; for example, oral lesions that could impact nutritional intake, diabetic control, and/or deter individuals from participating in communal nutritional breaks and thus negatively impacting socialization. In addition to unattended pain found with oral lesions, decreased quality of life, loneliness and depression may coexist.

The appreciation of the human emotional and economic toll caused by aging and chronic diseases has caused agencies to attempt improvements to the functional years of life through health care advances. The development of evidence-based, clinical practice guidelines is an effort to optimize the treatment of chronic diseases such as hypertension or coronary artery disease. Most commonly, these guidelines have a singular disease focus, not considering the impact of other possible comorbidities.[6] When diseases are treated as stand-alone, overtreatment is likely.[7] The input of an interdisciplinary team thus becomes vitally important to manage these medically complex patients; involving other professionals from the entire health system spectrum helps to minimize overtreatment and provides a more appropriate holistic approach.

In addition, clinical practice guidelines are not generally constructed with the patient at the center, often focusing on immediate medical or physiologic concerns with little notice of barriers that might impede the actions recommended by the guidelines, assessment of changes in overall functionality, or consideration of the patients' or caregivers' concerns.[8] For older adults, clinical practice guidelines need to be centered on the multiplicity of findings often seen in older patients and on efforts to promote coordinated care across clinicians and settings. Owing to the current lack of these systems, fragmentation, inefficiencies, and increased costs result from clinical practice guideline use.[9]

Dentistry has few clinical practice guidelines, with those that do exist (eg, prophylactic antibiotic use for certain cardiac[10] or joint replacement conditions),[11] also placing the disease at the center rather than the patient's and family's goals, as recommended by the National Quality Forum.[11] Nor has dentistry created clinical practice guidelines that cross disciplines and consider the intersection of chronic systemic disease with oral health conditions and psychosocial issues. Yet, those with systemic multimorbidities are more likely to seek dental care than those without this finding;[12] a number of studies have demonstrated high morbidity relationships, especially in the edentulous patient.[13]

Treatment Implications

It is in the patient's best interest for oral health care practitioners to prepare to care for more older adults with multiple chronic systemic diseases, more episodes of oral disease, and interposing psychosocial influencing variables. There are multiple conditions seen in older adults that can present with similar phenotypes. For this reason, in this article, we take a broad approach, presenting various common phenotypes and including examples of oral findings and oral treatment implications for each topic.

INFECTION AND INFLAMMATION

Immunosenescence describes changes in the immune system's capability that occur with advancing age in the absence of disease; such changes normally cause only modest decreases in immune function. This impact becomes more substantial when other conditions coexist (eg, malnutrition, diabetes, human immunodeficiency virus, etc). When dysfunction is severe, autoimmunity, diminished surveillance capability, and increased susceptibility to infections arise.[14]

Even when inflammation is low grade, it has an effect on aging. "Inflammaging" describes this proinflammatory state, considered to be a proxy marker and influencer of aging progression. Inflammaging impacts disease susceptibility, is a part of multimorbidities such as frailty, and causes an overall lessening of physical, cognitive, and life span capabilities.[15] **Fig. 1** displays the relationship between lifespan aging and inflammation.[16] If inflammation occurs in the short term, it is part of the body's natural defense mechanism and causes no lasting effects; however, when a source of infection and inflammation is prolonged, such as is seen with periodontal disease and caries, systemic diseases (eg, atherosclerosis, diabetes, kidney failure, and neurodegenerative disorders including Alzheimer disease) are negatively impacted.[15]

In addition to chronic conditions, intraoral bacteria can also directly cause serious acute systemic infections, such as endocarditis, brain abscesses, septic arthritis, and infections of joints and bone, and increase the risk for aspiration pneumonia,[17] yet another reason to eliminate any intraoral inflammation. Exposure to infectious agents causes inflammation that can influence the progression of atherosclerosis; periodontal treatment to remove inflammation could diminish the risk of myocardial infarction and stroke in older adults.[16] Epidemiologic evidence also links periodontal disease with diabetes and predisposes patients with diabetes to periodontal disease.[16]

Older adults have high rates of autoimmunity, when the individual's own antibodies (autoantibodies) act as foreign antigens, attacking serosal surfaces, joints, eyes, and/or skin at the molecular, cellular, or tissue levels. Examples of autoimmune conditions seen more commonly in elders include pernicious anemia, thyroiditis, bullous pemphigoid, rheumatoid arthritis, and temporal arteritis.[14] Some autoimmune conditions may present with aphthous type oral ulcerations and chronic jaw osteomyelitis.[18] Chronic inflammation can generate an immunosuppressive microenvironment that provides further advantages for tumor formation and progression.[19]

Treatment Implications

In an effort to eliminate acute and low-grade inflammation from the oral cavity, more vigilance and at times more aggressive treatment may be needed against periodontal conditions and caries. A customized approach for each individual should be based on the individual's presentation of disease and a thorough assessment of his or her

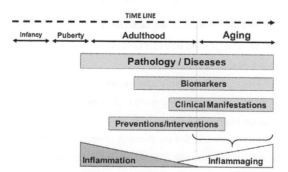

Fig. 1. Relationship of inflammaging to timeline events. (*From* Fulop T, Witkowski JM, Olivieri F, et al. The integration of inflammaging in age-related diseases. Semin Immunol. 2018;40:22; with permission. (Figure 3 in original).)

unique strengths and capabilities, as well as considerations of the family's and/or caregiver's roles, capacities, and interests. **Box 1** displays elements of preventive plans for older adults.

Typically, ongoing surveillance of intraoral infection should not ignore systemic signs such as fever. When challenged, however, the aging immune system is not always capable of demonstrating fever. Therefore, assessing and monitoring body temperature changes over multiple visits and comparing readings with that person's baseline value may provide better information on any temperature elevations than a standardized normal temperature target.

NUTRITION AND MALNUTRITION

Malnutrition describes a state of nutrition whereby a deficiency of nutrients results in changes to the body (shape, size, and composition), and its functional capabilities that is, clinically obvious. Early detection of malnutrition is difficult owing to multiple, conflicting criteria and, as a result, it frequently becomes advanced before being noticed. When finally diagnosed, malnutrition is still not always properly addressed, even though it has been clearly shown to be a factor associated with morbidity, mortality, and cost of care.[20,21]

The prevalence of malnutrition in older adults is complex and multidirectional, stemming from different operating domains (eg, oral, psychosocial, physical, lifestyle, health, and eating habits), all of which influence each other. These domains vary from person to person and over time and are cohort anchored, being higher in older adults with multimorbidities especially when health deterioration, lack of physical activity and dependency in the activities of daily living (ADLs) are present.[22] The relationships between factors correlated with malnutrition in older adults can be seen in a graphic at the following website (https://nutritionandaging.org/wp-content/uploads/2017/01/DetermineNutritionChecklist.pdf) that can be easily used by the dental practitioner and staff to instruct patients and family members or care givers and can also be used as a self-help home reminder.[23]

Malnutrition also seems to have multiple effects on the oral tissues and subsequent oral disease. Conditions such as recurrent aphthous stomatitis, atrophic glossitis, or a painful, burning tongue characterized by inflammation and defoliation are possibly caused by nutritional deficiencies such as vitamin B and iron. A lack of protein and deficiencies of certain micronutrients such as vitamins, zinc, and iron can

---

Box 1
Strategies to discourage inflammation in the oral cavity

- Risk assessment for diseases of hard and soft tissues
- Evaluation of physical plaque removal skills
- Recommendation of manual and/or electronic devices
- Possible caregiver assistance in managing daily oral hygiene
- Demonstrated ongoing improved daily oral hygiene
- Preventing caries and periodontal disease through chemopreventive agents
- Selection of in office and at home adjuncts to mechanical cleaning
- Replacement of saliva with appropriate substitutes
- Development of regular professional recare plan

influence the amount and the composition of the saliva, limiting its protective properties.[24]

The systematic review performed by O'Keeffe and colleagues[25] provides moderate evidence that chewing difficulties, mouth pain, gum issues, multimorbidity, visual and hearing impairments, smoking status, alcohol consumption, physical activity levels, and even complaints about taste of food and specific nutrient intakes were not correlated with malnutrition; there is low-quality evidence that loss of interest in life, access to Meals on Wheels, and modified texture diets are determinants of malnutrition. Further, the influence of some potential determinants of malnutrition such as dental status, swallowing, cognitive function, depression, residential status, medication intake and/or polypharmacy, constipation, and periodontal disease were conflicting.[25] Additional research in this area is needed because malnutrition is strongly associated with sarcopenia, which may impact periodontal disease, support of complete dentures, and frailty.

Treatment Implications

The Determine Your Nutritional Health is an easy and brief (10 question) survey to which the patient can be introduced and can self-administer in just a few minutes in the dental office. Its answers provide important insights into the patient's nutritional behaviors as well as several other areas including the impact of the dentition on eating, weight loss, and the patient's ability to manage multiple ADLs and instrumental ADLs as related to food preparation and consumption. Patients with difficulties highlighted by this survey can then be referred to the local Area Agencies on Aging offices for help in finding state and local resources that can include nutritional information programs as well as food distribution programs. The survey is available at the previously mentioned website:

https://nutritionandaging.org/wp-content/uploads/2017/01/DetermineNutritionChecklist.pdf [22]

WEIGHT LOSS

Unintentional weight loss (10 lbs. in the past year) occurs in 15% to 20% of people older than 65 years of age and is related to increased risk for morbidity and mortality. There is a higher prevalence of this finding in nursing home residents (50%–60%) as compared with community-dwelling elders (27%).[26]

Unintentional weight loss can be a result of decreased intake (the most common explanation in older adults), increased nutrient loss owing to malabsorption, and excess systemic demands resulting from malignancies. Weight loss may also be associated with depression and dementia. Community-dwelling elders may become unable physically and/or cognitively to grocery shop and cook meals or have limited income or access to nutritional foods. Certain medications can cause anorexia. Conditions that impact the respiratory system such as emphysema, make the coordination of breathing and eating activities difficult; Sjogren's syndrome may decrease the selection of a variety of foods owing to a self-recognition of an inadequate amount of saliva to prepare the bolus of food for swallowing.

Besides oral conditions influencing weight loss, it is also possible that the anorexia of aging may be at work. A decrease in lean body mass, bone mass, and the basal metabolic rate, coupled with a decrease in the senses of taste and smell and altered gastric signals leading to early satiation combine to bring about this effect. The resulting weight loss is very gradual, a little less than one-half of a pound a year.[27]

Oral health has often been described as one of the factors affecting weight in older adults; aspects such as teeth and denture-related issues, oral pain, oral lesions, dry mouth, and periodontal problems can prevent masticatory function, resulting in an imbalanced diet. Oral health often deteriorates during aging, sometimes owing to morbidities or behaviors, for example, poor oral hygiene or smoking. Dry mouth can negatively impact the taste and texture perception of food.[28] Recently, Kiesswetter and colleagues[29] found that community-dwelling elders self-reported estimation of their own oral status significantly correlated to their clinical body weight. Perhaps this one question could be easily integrated into clinical practice to identify older people at risk of weight loss and to initiate oral interventions.

Treatment Implications

Given the high prevalence of the anorexia of aging, it is likely that some family members concerned that weight loss could be related to a lack of/or ill-fitting dentures or other dentition related problems will bring their aging relatives who have lost weight to the dental office. A thorough examination, especially of the fit of prostheses, is needed because there may or may not be any deficiencies for the dentist to repair.

When weight loss does occur, it often results in the loosening of dentures, friction sores on the edentulous ridges, dissatisfaction with the fit, and ultimately decreases in life satisfaction. Unintentional weight loss caught early and investigated may allow early diagnosis and reversal of morbid trends. Consider adding height and weight assessments to the regular collection of vital signs, especially for your older adult patients to track insidious weight loss.

MUSCLE WEAKNESS

Muscle weakness can be the result of the combined effects of sarcopenia, osteopenia, and organopenia. Whereas sarcopenia is the loss of muscle mass as an outcome of normal aging, osteopenia describes the depletion over time of bone mass owing to an imbalance between resorptive and formative processes,[30] with organopenia being the loss in appendicular muscle and bone mass with increasing age.[31] All of these conditions contribute to the increasing prevalence of disability in older adults.

In sarcopenia, the rate of muscle loss ranges between 1% and 2% per year at ages greater than 50 years, with 25% of people less than 70 years of age and 40% of those greater than 80 years of age being sarcopenic. When existing alone, sarcopenia is likely a minor and modifiable risk factor for health outcomes, but not when found in conjunction with declining muscle strength and physical functioning. A sedentary lifestyle and bed rest often result in microcirculatory disturbances in the skeletal muscle, atrophy, protein loss, and so on, resulting in decreases in muscle mass, structure, and strength.[32]

Muscle weakness results from declinations of both neurologic and muscular dynamics, or dynapenia that recognizes the force-generating capacity of the skeletal muscles as a component.[33] Muscle weakness also contributes to dysfunctions of locomotion and balance in the elderly with vitamin D deficiency playing a significant role; more than one-half of all women treated for osteoporosis in the United States and Europe are estimated to have low levels as a result of decreased dietary intake, diminished sunlight exposure, decreased skin thickness, impaired intestinal absorption, and impaired hydroxylation in the liver and kidneys.[34] **Fig. 2** presents an overview of the interplay between poor oral status, malnutrition, and sarcopenia.[35]

Vitamin D is important to calcium absorption in the gastrointestinal tract with adequate levels decreasing the risk of fractures. Even when taken uncoupled with

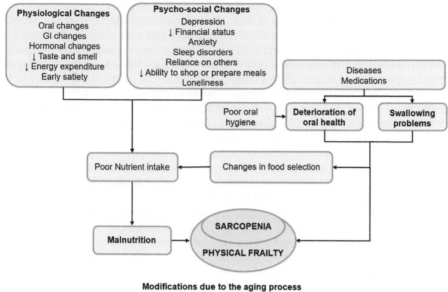

Fig. 2. Overview of the interplay between poor oral status, malnutrition, and sarcopenia. GI, gastrointestinal. (*From* Azzolino D, Passarelli PC, De Angelis P, et al. Poor oral health as a determinant of malnutrition and sarcopenia. Nutrients. 2019;11:2898. (CC BY 4.0 Open Access License).)

calcium, vitamin D shows improvement in osteoporosis. Some researchers have found a relationship between vitamin D, and periodontal disease.[36] Although not a causal factor, Megson and colleagues[37] suggest that decreased bone mineral density and periodontitis have shared risk factors.

Overall, the gradual loss of muscle strength below a certain threshold results in functional impairment, the need for assistance in the performance of ADLs, and increased risk of falling and nonvertebral fractures.[32] It is possible that grip strength and upper arm strength are associated, especially in the poststroke patient.[38] Paresis can result in 1-sided loss of muscle strength of the upper extremity on the contralateral stroke side, decreasing the ability to use the arm and hand fully. If the affected side was dominant, the patient can have a great deal of difficulty retraining the nondominant hand for usual ADL tasks.

Treatment Implications

Because oral home care is highly dependent on upper arm strength and hand grip to use various dental cleaning devices, the preservation of muscle strength in older adults is critical and rehabilitation of upper limb capabilities in a stroke patient is of paramount importance. Patients can be shown procedural modifications in how to use implements that minimize the impact of their losses. For example, sitting at a table and propping one's elbows on the tabletop as oral hygiene devices are being used helps to override the muscular weaknesses of the upper extremity. The tabletop can also serve as an anchor to the pivot points (elbows) when both hands are needed to jointly guide the toothbrush or flossing device to the mouth from the tabletop-elbow prop. Using this strategy can also offset the negative factor of weight of a battery powered toothbrush.

In dental practice, we typically do not have dynamometers to measured grip strength, but a general impression of such strength can be judged in the dental practice by introducing oneself to the patient, accompanied by a handshake. If a patient is unable to grasp another's hand and hold it, or does so only weakly, some thoughtful planning is needed in developing a doable oral health care home program. Handle diameters sized at 30 to 40 mm are the most comfortable,[39] in contrast with that of 10 to 15 mm (the size of manual toothbrushes). Therefore, enlargement of the toothbrush handle or recommending a battery-operated toothbrush should be considered.

Here is a good example of why an interdisciplinary team approach is so important to older adults: the poststroke dental patient is likely to continue to benefit from the guidance of a physical therapist in regaining strength and function even after the immediate poststroke rehabilitation period, as well as an occupational therapist who can assess and recommend methods and instrumentation to aid in meeting ADLs, even when diminished physical functioning remains.

Encouraging the patient at every dental appointment to continue performing the exercises learned during poststroke rehabilitation or in any number of exercise classes for healthy aging seniors needs to be a part of a lifelong daily routine. Exercise is important to the continuous training, retraining, restoring, and maintaining of muscular strength to perform activities throughout the lifespan, including those for managing one's own oral hygiene.

FALLS

Falls are the leading cause of fatal and nonfatal injuries in people aged 65 or older. Even in community-dwelling older adults, the fall rate can be as high as 75% over a 3-month interval,[40] with 45% of the falls resulting in injuries, 25% of which are likely to be bone fracture.[41] Although an intrinsic lack of bone integrity owing to structural skeletal losses (eg, osteoporosis) plays a role in the skeletal damage sustained in a fall, bone malignancies, and treatments with radiation and hormonal therapy among other medications may also be contributors. Nonskeletal influences of falls include fatigue, peripheral neuropathy, dizziness, and sensory disorders of vision and balance. Those who have fallen previously are more likely to fall again as the underlying cause is often not corrected or correctable. Trauma to the face as a result of falls may include abrasions, ecchymosis, and fractures. Similar intraoral findings include lacerations of the tongue and lips, and possible damage to the dentition. Because cuts and bruises are one of the signs of elder abuse, when such damage is observed, a full history of injuries should be taken by the provider to distinguish whether a report should be filed with the proper governmental agency. **Box 2** presents some approaches to preventing decline and improving muscle strength and coordination.[42]

Treatment Implications

When elder abuse is suspected and it is unknown if the state or local government has an Elder Abuse Hotline, login to the State Resources Section of the National Center on Elder Abuse website at https://eldercare.acl.gov/Public/Resources/LearnMoreAbout/Elder_Rights.aspx#Abuse [43] and use the resources and instructions to fulfill your duties as mandated reporters of elder abuse.

With the falls rate in older adults increasing, the Centers for Disease Control and Prevention through its STEADI initiative has recommended that all health care providers participate in helping to stem the tide. A suite of information including videos and other educational material is available on the STEADI website https://www.cdc.gov/steadi/about.html.[44] Dental practitioners can help identify individuals at risk by

---

Box 2
Integrative approaches to preventing decline and improving muscle strength and coordination

Diet
  Mediterranean diet, anti-inflammatory diet (include fatty fish, more vegetables and fruits), increased carotenoid intake, soy.

Exercise
  Promote mobility, walking, resistance training, yoga, tai chi, comprehensive fall prevention programs.

Supplements
  Fish oil, vitamin D, whey protein, soy protein, and soy isoflavones, amino acid supplementation; anti-inflammatory herbs like curcumin, if general inflammation is present or suspected; the role of vitamin E is not clear.

Androgens and testosterone
  Only if deficiency state is present after careful assessment of risk; not recommended for routine use.

From Kogan M, Cheng S, Rao S, et al. Integrative medicine for geriatric and palliative care. Med Clin North Am. 2017;101(5):1010; with permission. (Table 1 in original).

---

asking 3 simple screening questions and referring for further assessment any older adults who say yes to any of the questions (**Box 3**).

There is much the dental health care provider can do to prevent falls in the dental office, beginning with a fall risk assessment for each patient and flagging those patients at the highest risk. An environmental assessment should include the approach to the dental office or clinic (walkway, garage access, elevator, steps or stairs) to ensure hazards are removed and lighting is adequate. Further preparing the dental office includes removing obstacles in hallways, ensuring even and smooth transitions across changing floor textures, installing handrails even when there are only 1 or 2 steps, and ensuring there is adequate lighting throughout the office. Remembering to sit the patient upright in the dental chair and insisting the patient stay in the chair for a minimum of 3 minutes after prolonged treatment in a supine position will stabilize the blood pressure, thus minimizing any potential falls from orthostatic hypotensive episodes that are often the adverse outcomes of so many medications with which older adults are being treated.

Box 3
Are you asking older adults patients the right questions?

When you see patients older than 65, make these 3 questions a routine part of your examination:
- Have you fallen in the past year?
- Do you feel unsteady when standing or walking?
- Do you worry about falling?

If your patient answers "yes" to any of these key screening questions, they are considered at increased risk of falling. A further assessment is recommended.

CDC STEADI Initiative for Health Care Providers to determine risk for falls. Available at: https://www.cdc.gov/steadi/index.html. Accessed July 25, 2020.

POLYPHARMACY

Polypharmacy, the consistent use of 5 or more prescription medications on a daily basis, has been found in 13% to 92% of older adults. Negative outcomes as a result of polypharmacy include drug–drug interactions and adverse events, often owing to physiologic changes seen with aging such as decreases in the detoxifying capabilities of the kidney and liver, changes in body muscle/fat ratios, and the negative influences of systemic disease, including comorbid conditions and their associated medications. The patients most likely to experience polypharmacy are those seeing multiple doctors and/or using several pharmacies who have concurrent conditions.[45] Certain patient populations such as older adults living with human immunodeficiency virus are also more likely to demonstrate polypharmacy.[46] As a result, dosing adjustments are frequently required. For older adults living with human immunodeficiency virus the risk for drug–drug interactions is especially great owing to the multidrug regimen needed to treat human immunodeficiency virus, as well as other medications to treat the conditions frequently seen in aging.[47]

Some medications being taken for systemic conditions in older adults can require significant adjustments to dental treatment protocols. For example, those on bisphosphonate or denosumab therapy for osteoporosis or certain cancer types may require much more caution and antibiotics when extractions or other procedures involving bone injury are contemplated or intraoral lesions are present owing to the risk of developing medication-related osteonecrosis of the jaws.[48] See **Fig. 3** for clinical photos and **Box 4** for summarized tips to minimize medication-related osteonecrosis of the jaws.

Newer medications being developed such as direct-acting oral anticoagulants have more predictable pharmacokinetics, shorter half-lives, and fewer food interactions,

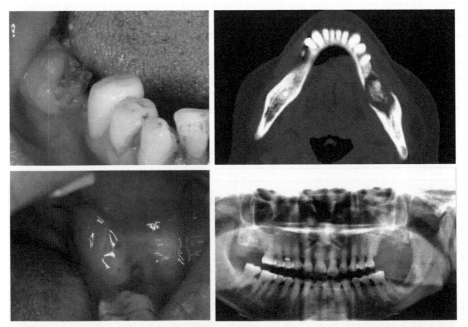

Fig. 3. Bisphosphonates. ("Pictures provided by the team from the Orofacial Pain/ Oral Medicine Program at USC" - With Permission.)

Box 4
Preventive tips for dentist treating patients taking bisphosphonates or denosumab

Before starting drug therapy
- Obtain a detailed medical history from the patient, family member, or physician.
- Thoroughly evaluate for any oral disease.
- Aggressively treat intraoral infection.
- Provide endodontic care for those teeth that can be saved.
- Extract any teeth with a poor prognosis.
- Complete any needed surgical procedures.
- Educate the patient on the need for vigilance in watching for oral lesions.

Once therapy has started
- Considered antibiotic prophylaxis before undertaking invasive dental care.
- Perform all procedures, including surgical, ones as atraumatically as possible.
- Be sure to achieve primary closure.
- Reinforce good oral hygiene techniques.
- Add chemotherapeutics as appropriate.
- Follow-up closely with your patients.
- Dentures should be assessed regularly and adjustments and relines provided.
- Provide instruction about the importance of denture hygiene and nighttime removal.
- Remind patients of the overall need for vigilance for lesions and return to care.

Adapted from Otto S, Pautke C, Van den Wyngaert T, et al. Medication-related osteonecrosis of the jaw: Prevention, diagnosis and management in patients with cancer and bone metastases. Cancer Treat Rev. 2018;69:183; with permission. (Boxes 1 and 2 in original).

---

requiring less monitoring, and making invasive dental procedures less risky for prolonged bleeding than warfarin. A cost analysis of the direct-acting oral anticoagulants has demonstrated decreased expense when managing patients with nonvalvular atrial fibrillation, so the expectation is that more older adults will be taking these newer drugs in the future.[49]

Treatment Implications

It is prudent for the practitioner to run the patient's medication profile along with any medications being considered for dental care, through an electronic drug information software program such as epocrates® or Lexicomp®. Doing so will display any drug–drug interactions, the type and rate of adverse effects for each, and recommendations for dosing adjustments for those who are older or have kidney or liver dysfunction. With the information gleaned, treatment adjustments can then be made based on the findings. **Table 1** displays some of the drug–drug interactions affecting the oral cavity.[50]

Performing drug inventories on the duration of usage, dose, specific medication, and delivery method are important for all medications being taken, because the risk of adverse events increases significantly with increasing numbers of drugs and doses. This practice may turn up some important irregularities in use, such as drug duplication (the patient is taking the same drug twice with one prescription bottle displaying the drug's generic name and another with the brand name). Some drugs (eg, bisphosphonates, denosumab, corticosteroids) require pretreatment planning before care delivery owing specifically to the drugs' adverse events.

HYPOSALIVARY FUNCTION

One of the most common adverse drug effects of polypharmacy is decreased salivary flow or salivary hypofunction, resulting in higher rates of dental caries, candidiasis,

Table 1
Common antihypertensive drug classes, dental side effects, and drug–drug interactions

Drug Class	Dental Side Effects	Common Drug Interactions
Beta-blockers	Dry mouth, taste changes, lichenoid reaction	NSAIDs, epinephrine, local anesthetics, bronchodilators, vasopressors
ACE inhibitors	Rash, dry cough, loss of taste, taste changes, dry mouth, ulceration, angioedema, burning mouth, lichenoid reactions, neutropenia, delayed healing, gingival bleeding	NSAIDs
Angiotensin II receptor blockers	Dry mouth, angioedema, sinusitis, taste loss, cough	Systemic antifungal, sedatives
Calcium channel blockers	Gingival enlargement, dry mouth, altered taste, erythema multiforme	Benzodiazepines, parenteral anesthetic agents, aspirin, NSAIDs, erythromycin, clarithromycin, cyp-3a4 concentrations
Alpha-blockers	Dry mouth, taste changes	NSAIDs, CNS depressants, salicylates
Diuretics	Dry mouth, lichenoid reaction, altered taste (acetazolamide)	NSAIDs, barbiturates, fluconazole
Direct-acting vasodilators	Facial flushing, gingival bleeding, infection, lapus-like oral/skin lesions, lymphadenopathy	NSAIDs, opioids
Central-acting agents	Dry mouth, sedation, taste changes, linenoid reactions (methyldopa), parotid pain, opioids	NSAIDs, sedatives, epinephrine
Combined alpha-/beta-blockers	Taste changes	Epinephrine, NSAIDs

Abbreviations: ACE, angiotensin-converting enzyme; NSAIDs, nonsteroidal anti-inflammatory drugs.
From Southerland JH, Gill DG, Gangula PR, et al. Dental management in patients with hypertension: challenges and solutions. Clin Cosmet Investig Dent. 2016;8:114; with permission.

halitosis, taste disturbance, and functional problems during chewing, speaking, and swallowing.[51] **Fig. 4** provides examples of the effect of inadequate saliva. Salivary hypofunction may have other causes including radiation therapy, autoimmune conditions, and primary salivary diseases; however, the treatment of salivary hypofunction demonstrates more similarities than differences. **Table 2** presents other causes of salivary hypofunction. There is no single product or strategy that has been determined to be the best for all, and patient preference is an important factor.[52]

Treatment Implications

Dehydration in older adults is a common and significant finding in patients with even small amounts (1%–2%) of body water deficiencies resulting in cognitive performance declines. Given that dry mouth signs and symptoms may be part of the whole body dehydration presentation, asking a patient to keep a fluid intake diary for as little as

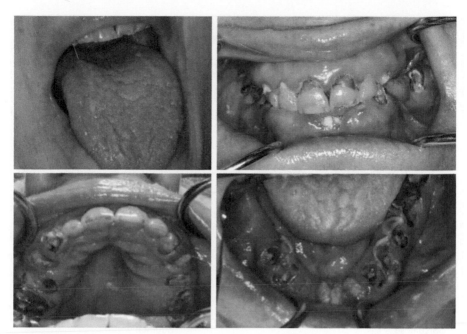

Fig. 4. Dry mouth and caries. ("Pictures provided by the team from the Roseann Mulligan Special Patients Clinic at USC" - With Permission.)

a few days helps them and you to see how much fluid is being consumed. Sometimes when intake is increased by just a small amount, the signs and symptoms of dry mouth may decrease or disappear.

If the patient's hyposalivation condition is severe, negotiating a change with the primary care physician and/or pharmacist to another medication that is less xerogenic or reducing the dose of the current one should be attempted. Unfortunately, many medications in the same drug class have similar xerogenic profiles, leaving few alternatives. Because there are a variety of strategies for treating dry mouth, one or more of them should be attempted, provided that they do not cause more harm. For example, increasing the flow through the use of sialogues (eg, lozenges, hard candies) that contain sugar are likely to cause caries and decrease control of blood glucose in patients with diabetes. More frequent follow-up professional visits are needed for care, including in-office fluoride applications in addition to increased home fluoride options. Although there are some medications that can be used to directly stimulate the glands (pilocarpine and cevimeline) owing to their high cholinergic effects, they must be used with caution in older adults with comorbid conditions.[53] With the abundance of options, care plans must be individualized so that the patient receives the relief being sought with the proper treatment modality. **Table 3** reviews different strategies for treatment of dry mouth.[52]

EDENTULISM

Oral health problems can actually begin at early ages and become chronic over time ultimately impacting the oral health of older adults. Because people are keeping their teeth longer, more oral disease is occurring as a result of years of risk accumulation, including that owing to poorly controlled chronic diseases and inadequate oral

Table 2 Etiology or causes of salivary gland hypofunction and xerostomia	
General	**Iatrogenic**
Old age	Medications[a]
Female sex	Therapeutic irradiation[a]
Dehydration	Chemotherapy/immunotherapy
Disability (cognitive and physical)	Chronic graft versus host disease
Institutionalization	Salivary duct ligation
Habits (mouth breathing, smoking, alcohol and drug abuse)	Liquid diet feeding
Compromised masticatory function	
Diseases	
Salivary gland diseases and disorders	Infections
Agenesis of the salivary glands	HIV/AIDS
(with or without ectodermal dysplasia)	Hepatitis C virus
Sia loadenitis	Tuberculosis
Sia lolithiasis	Human T lymphotropic virus
Chronic inflammatory autoimmune diseases	Psychogenic diseases and conditions
Sjogren's syndrome[a]	Stress
Other rheumatologic diseases; rheumatoid	Anxiety and nervousness
arthritis, SLE, scleroderma, mixed connective	Depression
tissue disease, etc	Eating disorders (anorexia nervosa,
Sarcoidosis	bulimia)
Amyloidosis	Others
Crohn's disease, ulcerative colitis	Cystic fibrosis
Endocrine diseases	Hypertension
Diabetes mellitus	Fibromyalgia
Hyperthyroidism and hypothyroidism	Chronic fatigue syndrome
Crushing syndrome	Burning mouth syndrome
Addison disease	Primary biliary cirrhosis
Neurologic diseases and disorders	Liver transplant candidates
Stroke	Renal diseases and Renal dialysis
Parkinson disease	Anemia
Bell's palsy	Atrophic gastritis
Alzheimer disease	

Abbreviation: HIV, human immunodeficiency virus.
  [a] Major causes of dry mouth.
  From Han P, Suarez-Durall P, Mulligan R. Dry mouth: a critical topic for older adult patients. J Prosthodont Res. 2015;59(1):10; with permission. (Table 1 in original).

hygiene. Unfortunately, a large variety of physical, psychological, and social issues often cause certain aging cohorts to access oral health care less frequently than younger groups. In particular, underserved racial/ethnic older adult groups are disproportionally impacted.[54] These findings suggest that more targeted oral health prevention and promotion activities in older adults are still needed across the spectrum of aging individuals.

A number of studies have demonstrated tooth loss to be associated with higher mortality, and not wearing dentures with poor quality of life and greater morbidity.[55] Infrequent cleaning of dentures or partials[56] and sleeping while wearing dentures resulted in a 1.3- and 2.3-fold increased risk of pneumonia, respectively.[57] Although the potential link between edentulism and mortality has not been shown to be causal, if saving or replacing teeth has the potential to contribute to an improved quality of life,

Table 3
Selective topical salivary stimulators, oral moisturizers and salivary substitutes for Dry Mouth signs and symptoms[a]

Preparation	Products	Active Ingredients
1. Saivary stimulators		
Sugarless chewing gums	Biotene dry mouth gum (GlaxoSmithKline)	Sorbitol, xylitol, maltitol
	Orbit (Wm. Wrigley Jr. Company)	Sorbitol, mannitol. xylitol
	Eclipse (Wm. Wrigley Jr. Company)	Maltitol, sorbitol, mannitol
	Extra (Wm. Wrigley Jr. Company)	Sorbitol, mannitol. maltitol
	Trident/Stimorol (Mondele z International)	Xylitol. sorbitol, mannitol
	Ice Breakers (The Hershey Company)	Xylitol
	Xylifresh (Leaf International)	Xylitol
	Spry Xylitol Gum (Spry Dental Defense System)	Xylitol, sorbitol
	Smint (Perfetti Van Melle)	Xylitol
Sugarless tablets/discs/ patches	Salix SST (Scandinavian Natural Health & Beauty Products. Inc)	Sorbitol, fruit acid
	Xylimelts (Orahealth Corporation)	Xylitol
Sugarless solution/spray	Mouth-Kote (Parnell Pharmaceuticals. Inc.)	Yerba santa, xylitol, lemon oil
Sugarless hard candy, mints, lozenges or lemon drops	Many preparations available	Sugar substitutes, citric acid, etc.
	Trident, Spry, Smint, ACT, etc.	
2. Oral moisturizers/salivary substitutes		
Mouth rinses/washes	Biotene Dry Mouth Oral Rinse (GlaxoSmithKline)	Glycerin, xylitol, sorbitol, propylene glycol, hydroxyethyl cellulose
	Colgate [1] Dry Mouth Relief Fluoride Mouthwash (Colgate)	Not available
	Spray Oral Rinse (Spry Dental Defense System)[a]	Xylitol, glycerin
	Oasis Moisturizing Mouth Wash (Oasis Consumer Healthcare)	Glycerin, water, sorbitol
	Act Total Care Dry Mouth Soothing Mouthwash (Chattem. Inc.)	Glycerin, sorbitol, xylitol, propylene glycol
Patches	Oramoist dry mouth Patches (Quantum)	Xylitol, polyvinylpyrrolidone, carbomer homopolymer, hydroxypropyl cellulose, lysozyme, lactoferrin
Spray	Water/Glycerine Spray	Glycerin
	MOI-STIR (Pendopharm. Pharmascience Inc.)	Carboxymethyicellulose sodium, giycerin
	Biotene Moisturizing Mouth Spray (GlaxoSmithKline)	Glycerin, xylitol, hydrogenated castor oil
	Oralube (Perrigo Australia)	Methyl hydroxybenzoate, sorbitol

(*continued on next page*)

Table 3
(continued)

Preparation	Products	Active Ingredients
	Spry Oral Mist (Spry Dental Defense System)	Glycerin, Xylitol, Sorbitol
	Oasis Moisturizing Mouth Spray (Oasis Consumer Healthcare)	Glycerin, sorbitol, poloxamer 338, PEG 60, hydrogenated castor oil
	CVS Dry Mouth Spray (CVS Pharmacy)/Rite Aid Dry Mouth Spray (Rite Aid Pharmacy)	Xylitol, aloe vera, lactoferrin, lyzozyme, glucoxidase, amylase, amylogucosidase, peptizyme
Gel	GC Dry Mouth Gel (GC America Inc.) Dentist dispensed	Not available
	Biotene Oral Balance Moisturizing Gel (GlaxoSmithKline)	Glycerin, sorbitol, xylitol, carbomer, hydroxyethyl cellulose
	Órajel Dry Mouth Gel (Church & Dwight. Inc.)	Glycerin
Toothpaste	Kotene Dry Mouth Fluoride Toothpaste (GlaxoSmithKline)	Glycerin, sorbitol
	Spry toothpaste (Spry Dental Defense System)	Glycerin, xylitol, sorbitol
Salivary substitute solution	Saliva Substitute (Roxane laboratories) Prescription	Purified water, sorbitol, sodium carboxymethyicellulose, etc.

This table is based on the information acquired from http://www.drymouth.info/practitioner/treatment.asp and web searches.

[a] Some products contain citric acid and alcohol, which can irritate the mucosa of patients with dry mouth. Many dry mouth products contain fluoride.

From; "Han P. Suarez-Durall P, Mulligan R. Dry mouth: a critical topic for older adult patients. J Prosthodont Res. 2015;59(1):6-19." with permission

better nutrition, and decreased mortality, it is incumbent that policies and clinical practice be implemented to correct this inequity.[47]

Treatment Implications

Wearing complete dentures can have adverse effects on the supporting tissues causing residual ridge resorption, angular cheilitis, traumatic ulcers, denture stomatitis, soft tissue hyperplasia, and temporomandibular disorders. These findings may have multifactorial causes, especially in the elderly, and usually can be easily managed. Overall, edentulous patients are satisfied with their complete dentures. Those who are not, require active listening from their providers, because psychological and emotional factors are extremely important when dealing with edentulous patients unhappy with their prostheses. Effective communication helps them to adapt to the dentures, thereby improving their quality of life.

COGNITIVE DECLINES

A frequently encountered condition seen when treating older adults is covert or frank signs of cognitive impairment, the prevalence of which is expected to double over the next 20 years.[49] Although some patients arrive at the dental office having already been diagnosed with a cognitive problem such as dementia, depression, past episodes of delusions, and so on, many others have not been diagnosed. In the early stages of mild cognitive impairment, it may be impossible for a practitioner to appreciate the subtleties of declining cognitive capabilities given the lack of previous or infrequent interactions with a particular patient and the capability of many older adults to compensate for their cognitive inadequacies after a lifetime of experiencing and navigating social environments.

Because a significant percentage (73.6%) of dentate adults 65 years of age or older make an annual visit to the dental office,[58] administering an informal cognitive screening is helpful for the practitioner to assess the patient's ability to understand the informed consent, participate in receiving care, make financial commitments, and follow through with aftercare recommendations. Collateral information obtained from accompanying family members can be useful in further learning of the patient's capabilities. Although there are a number of cognitive screening instruments available, one that takes little time to administer, but is sensitive in detecting mild cognitive impairment is the Montreal Cognitive Assessment.[49]

In a systematic review of the literature that investigated the association between cognitive status as recorded by various cognitive function tests and mastication, poorer mastication was determined to be a significant risk factor for having dementia or mild memory impairment.[59]

Treatment Implications

It is not necessary to use a formal assessment instrument to perform a cognitive assessment in the dental office. The discerning practitioner begins to assess the patient at the moment of the first encounter, observing the patient's appearance and grooming, posture, behavior, orientation to his or her surroundings, speech volume and choice of words, ambulation ability, and so on. Guiding the interview through topics of significance to the patient's life or in current events' news could also gauge the patient's memory and reliability as an accurate historian. Being aware of any limitations to the patient's visual or hearing capabilities and past occupational and educational level attainments and literacy are also important because these factors have an impact on cognitive attainment. It is important to ask patients questions that are open ended, requiring them to use a variety of higher cognitive skills to formulate answers and express themselves. For those unable to do so, consultations with family members and possibly the patient's physician about the patient's abilities are likely needed.

SUMMARY

It is well-understood that many older adults have multiple morbidities that can impact their oral, systemic, and psychological health and in turn are affected by additional factors such as treatment regimens for their morbidities as well as environmental, cultural, social supports and cohesion, and personal factors and behaviors. Each variable and its strength in the patient's life must be considered to develop an appropriate care delivery strategy that weighs the extent of all influencing variables. By assessing the common phenotypic presentations of older adults, we can better understand, select, and coordinate involving colleagues from an interdisciplinary team on the treatment modifications that are needed to navigate and deliver the most appropriate care for our older adult patients in an individualized, strategic, and successful manner.

CLINICS CARE POINTS

- When physiologic aging is combined with comorbidities, negative impacts on health become highly evident.
- Treating patients with comorbidities often requires preplanning, so that modifications to usual care routines are made before providing dental treatment.
- Consultation with the patient's primary physician may be needed.
- Prepare to care for more older adults with multiple chronic systemic diseases, more episodes of oral disease, and interposing psychosocial influencing variables.
- Be more vigilant about eliminating acute and low-grade inflammation from the oral cavity.
- Compensate for the loss of strength in the upper arms and hands when designing oral home care.
- Show your patients procedural techniques in how to use oral hygiene implements that minimize the impact of their losses.
- Encourage older patients to continue rehabilitation or lifelong exercise programs to maintain motor strength, including that of the upper limbs.
- Be an active health care participant in the Centers for Disease Control and Prevention's STEADI initiative to decrease falls experienced by older adults.
- Assess the dental office, including the associated parking area, elevator, stairs, and treatment rooms, for environmental hazards that could contribute to falls.
- Use an electronic medication assessment program such as epocrates or Lexicomp to check the potential for any dental medications to cause drug–drug interactions or adverse reactions with the patient's current medication regimen.
- Neither stop nor alter the dose of direct-acting oral anticoagulants before dental procedures because the risk of stopping them outweighs the consequences of prolonged bleeding that can be managed by external or local measures.
- When dry mouth is present, recommending a short interval (2- or 3-day) fluid intake diary is valuable; if a deficiency is noted, plan cautious increases of water while concurrently reassessing any changes in dry mouth signs and/or symptoms.
- Consider adding height and weight assessments to the regular collection of vital signs, especially for older adult patients, because an early diagnosis of unintentional weight loss allows for reversal of morbid trends.
- Effective communication helps edentulous patients to better adapt to the dentures, thereby improving their quality of life.

DISCLOSURE

Dr Mulligan and Dr Suarez attest that they have no commercial or financial conflicts of interest related to the contents of this article.

REFERENCE

1. World Health Organization [homepage on the Internet]. Facts about ageing. 2014. Available at: http://www.who.int/ageing/about/facts/en/. Accessed June 27, 2020.
2. Available at: http://www.cdc.gov/chronicdisease/resources/publications/aag/pdf/2011/healthy_aging_aag_508.pdf. Accessed June 27, 2020.

3. Bell SP, Saraf AA. Epidemiology of multimorbidity in older adults with cardiovascular disease. Clin Geriatr Med 2016;32(2):215–26.
4. Lewis A, Kitson A, Harvey G. Improving oral health for older people in the home care setting: an exploratory implementation study. Australas J Ageing 2016;35(4): 273–328.
5. Sinnige J, Braspenning J, Schellevis F, et al. The prevalence of disease clusters in older adults with multiple chronic diseases–a systematic literature review. PLoS One 2013;8(11):e79641.
6. Upshur RE, Tracy S. Chronicity and complexity: is what's good for the diseases always good for the patients? Can Fam Physician 2008;54(12):1655–8.
7. Cesari M, Marzetti E, Canevelli M, et al. Geriatric syndromes: how to treat. Virulence 2017;8(5):577–85.
8. Mutasingwa DR, Ge H, Upshur RE. How applicable are clinical practice guidelines to elderly patients with comorbidities? Can Fam Physician 2011;57(7): e253–62.
9. National quality forum NQF: MCC measurement framework. Available at: https://www.qualityforum.org/Projects/Multiple_Chronic_Conditions_Measurement_Framework.aspx. Accessed July 26, 2020.
10. Wilson W, Taubert KA, Gewitz M, et al. Prevention of infective endocarditis: guidelines from the American Heart Association [published correction appears in Circulation. 2007 Oct 9;116(15):e376-7]. Circulation 2007;116(15):1736–54.
11. Sollecito TP, Abt E, Lockhart PB, et al. The use of prophylactic antibiotics prior to dental procedures in patients with prosthetic joints: evidence-based clinical practice guideline for dental practitioners—a report of the American dental association council on scientific affairs. J Am Dent Assoc 2015;146:11.
12. Wade A, Hobbs M, Green MA. Investigating the relationship between multimorbidity and dental attendance: a cross-sectional study of UK adults. Br Dent J 2019;226(2):138–43.
13. Islas-Granillo H, Borges-Yañez SA, Navarrete-Hernández JJ, et al. Indicators of oral health in older adults with and without the presence of multimorbidity: a cross-sectional study. Clin Interv Aging 2019;14:219–24.
14. Tummala MK, Taub DD, Ershler WB. Clinical immunology: immune senescence and the acquired immunodeficiency of aging. In: Fillet HM, Rockwood K, Young J, et al, editors. Brocklehurst's textbook of geriatric medicine and gerontology. 8th edition. Philadelphia: Elsevier; 2017. p. 781–8.e6.
15. Bektas A, Schurman SH, Sen R, et al. Aging, inflammation and the environment. Exp Gerontol 2018;105:10–8.
16. Fulop T, Witkowski JM, Olivieri F, et al. The integration of inflammaging in age-related diseases. Semin Immunol 2018;40:22, with permission.
17. Scannapieco FA, Cantos A. Oral inflammation and infection, and chronic medical diseases: implications for the elderly. Periodontol 2000 2016;72(1):153–75.
18. Scully C, Hodgson T, Lachmann H. Auto-inflammatory syndromes and oral health. Oral Dis 2008;14(8):690–9.
19. Wang D, DuBois RN. Immunosuppression associated with chronic inflammation in the tumor microenvironment. Carcinogenesis 2015;36(10):1085–93.
20. Abizanda P, Sinclair A, Barcons V, et al. Costs of malnutrition in institutionalized and community-dwelling older adults: a systematic review. J Am Med Dir Assoc 2016;17(1):17e23.
21. Sorbye LW, Schroll M, Finne Soveri H, et al. Unintended weight loss in the elderly living at home: the aged in Home Care Project (AdHOC). J Nutr Health Aging 2008;12(1):10e6.

22. Cereda E, Pedrolli C, Klersy C, et al. Nutritional status in older persons according to healthcare setting: a systematic review and meta-analysis of prevalence data using MNA®. Clin Nutr 2016;35(6):1282e90.
23. Available at: https://nutritionandaging.org/wp-content/uploads/2017/01/DetermineNutritionChecklist.pdf. Accessed October 30, 2020.
24. Sheetal Aparna, Hiremath Vinay Kumar, Patil Anand G, et al. Malnutrition and its oral outcome – a review. J Clin Diagn Res 2013;7(1):178–80.
25. O'Keeffe M, Kelly M, O'Herlihy E, et al. Potentially modifiable determinants of malnutrition in older adults: a systematic review. Clin Nutr 2019;38(6):2477–98.
26. Alibhai SMH, Greenwood C, Payette H. An approach to the management of unintentional weight loss in the elderly. CMAJ 2005;172:773–8.
27. Wallace JI, Schwartz RS. Epidemiology of weight loss in humans with special reference to wasting in the elderly. Int J Cardiol 2002;85:15–21.
28. Carlsson GE. Clinical morbidity and sequelae of treatment with complete dentures. J Prosthet Dent 1998;79(1):17–23.
29. Kiesswetter E, Keijser BJF, Volkert D, et al. Association of oral health with body weight: a prospective study in community-dwelling older adults. Eur J Clin Nutr 2020;74(6):961–9.
30. Otomo-Corgel J. Osteoporosis and osteopenia: implications for periodontal and implant therapy. Periodontol 2000 2012;59(1):111–39.
31. Manini TM. Organopenia. J Appl Physiol (1985) 2009;106(6):1759–60.
32. Seene T, Kaasik P. Muscle weakness in the elderly: role of sarcopenia, dynapenia, and possibilities for rehabilitation. Eur Rev Aging Phys Act 2012;9:109–17.
33. Clark BC, Manini TM. Functional consequences of sarcopenia and dynapenia in the elderly. Curr Opin Clin Nutr Metab Care 2010;13:271–6.
34. Janssens B, Petrovic M, Jacquet W, et al. Medication Use and Its Potential Impact on the Oral Health Status of Nursing Home Residents in Flanders (Belgium). J Am Med Dir Assoc 2017;18(9):809.e1–8.
35. Azzolino D, Passarelli PC, De Angelis P, et al. Poor oral health as a determinant of malnutrition and sarcopenia. Nutrients 2019;11:2898.
36. Jabbar S, Drury J, Fordham J, et al. Plasma vitamin D and cytokines in periodontal disease and postmenopausal osteoporosis. J Periodontal Res 2011;46:97–104.
37. Megson E, Kapellas K, Bartold PM. Relationship between periodontal disease and osteoporosis. Int J Evid Based Healthc 2010;8:129–39.
38. Ekstrand E, Lexell J, Brogårdh C. Grip strength is a representative measure of muscle weakness in the upper extremity after stroke. Top Stroke Rehabil 2016;23(6):400–5.
39. Kong YK, Lowe BD. Optimal cylindrical handle diameter for grip force tasks. Int J Ind Ergon 2005;35(Issue 6):495–507.
40. Overcash JA, Rivera HR Jr. Physical performance evaluation of older cancer patients: a preliminary study. Crit Rev Oncol Hematol 2008;68:233–41.
41. Sattar S, Alibhai SMH, Spoelstra SL, et al. The assessment, management, and reporting of falls, and the impact of falls on cancer treatment in community- dwelling older patients receiving cancer treatment: results from a mixed-methods study. J Geriatr Oncol 2019;10:98–104.
42. Kogan M, Cheng S, Rao S, et al. Integrative medicine for geriatric and palliative care. Med Clin North Am 2017;101(5):1010, with permission.
43. Available at: https://eldercare.acl.gov/Public/Resources/LearnMoreAbout/Elder_Rights.aspx#Abuse. Accessed on October 30, 2020.

44. Available at: https://www.cdc.gov/steadi/about.html. Accessed on October 30, 2020.
45. Lees J, Chan A. Polypharmacy in elderly patients with cancer: clinical implications and management. Lancet Oncol 2011;12(13):1249–57.
46. Guaraldi G, Malagoli A, Calcagno A, et al. The increasing burden and complexity of multi-morbidity and polypharmacy in geriatric HIV patients: a cross-sectional study of people aged 65 - 74 years and more than 75 years. BMC Geriatr 2018;18(1):99.
47. Guaraldi G, Milic J, Mussini C. Aging with HIV. Curr HIV/AIDS Rep 2019;16: 475–81.
48. Otto S, Pautke C, Van den Wyngaert T, et al. Medication-related osteonecrosis of the jaw: prevention, diagnosis and management in patients with cancer and bone metastases. Cancer Treat Rev 2018;69:177–87.
49. Amin A, Bruno A, Trocio J, et al. Comparison of differences in medical costs when new oral anticoagulants are used for the treatment of patients with non-valvular atrial fibrillation and venous thromboembolism vs warfarin or placebo in the US. J Med Econ 2015;18(6):399–409.
50. Southerland JH, Gill DG, Gangula PR, et al. Dental management in patients with hypertension: challenges and solutions. Clin Cosmet Investig Dent 2016;8:114, with permission.
51. Villa A, Wolff A, Aframian D, et al. World workshop on oral medicine VI: a systematic review of medication-induced salivary gland dysfunction: prevalence, diagnosis, and treatment. Clin Oral Investig 2015;19(7):1563–80.
52. Han P, Suarez-Durall P, Mulligan R. Dry mouth: a critical topic for older adult patients. J Prosthodont Res 2015;59(1):14.
53. Barbe AG. Medication-induced xerostomia and hyposalivation in the elderly: culprits, complications, and management. Drugs Aging 2018;35:877–85.
54. Dye BA, Weatherspoon DJ, Lopez-Mitnik G. Tooth loss among older adults according to poverty status in the United States from 1999 through 2004 and 2009 through 2014. J Am Dent Assoc 2019;150(1):9–23.
55. Gupta A, Felton DA, Jemt T, et al. Rehabilitation of edentulism and mortality: a systematic review. J Prosthodont 2019;28(5):526–35.
56. Kusama T, Aida J, Yamamoto T, et al. Infrequent denture cleaning increased the risk of pneumonia among community-dwelling older adults: a population-based cross-sectional study. Sci Rep 2019;9(1):13734.
57. Wittink MN, Pawar N, Martinez AP. Chapter 21 cognitive assessment in Fulmer T. and Chernof B. Handbook of geriatric assessment ed. 5th 2019 Jones and Bartlett learning. Available at: https://www.r2library.com/Resource/Title/1284144305/ch0021s0248.
58. CDC dental care among adults aged 65 and over. 2017. Available at: https://www.cdc.gov/nchs/products/databriefs/db337.htm#:~:text=In%202017%2C%20among%20adults%20aged%2065%20and%20over%2C%2065.6%25,those%20aged%2085%20and0over. Accessed July 27.2020.
59. Tada A, Miura H. Association between mastication and cognitive status: a systematic review. Arch Gerontol Geriatr 2017;70:44–53.

Poor Oral Health in the Etiology and Prevention of Aspiration Pneumonia

Frank A. Scannapieco, DMD, PhD

KEYWORDS

- Mouth • Pneumonia • Respiratory infection • Lungs • Oral microbiome
- Dental plaque • Biofilm

KEY POINTS

- The role of the oral microbiota in aspiration pneumonia (AP)—and the role of oral care in limiting it—is now well-recognized, because the bacteria that contribute to disease initiation often are aspirated from the oral cavity.
- Most cases of AP likely are the result of mixed infections involving 2 or more bacterial species, which may be more virulent than infections caused by a single species.
- Major risk factors for AP are those that undermine swallowing function and oral hygiene as well as underlying medical conditions that reduce immune function.
- Bacteria that colonize the teeth and other oral surfaces serve as a reservoir for respiratory pathogen colonization.
- Overall, oral cleansing protocols have been shown to reduce pneumonia in both edentulous and dentate subjects.

INTRODUCTION/HISTORY/DEFINITIONS/BACKGROUND

Pneumonia is an inflammatory condition of the lung parenchyma initiated by aspirated microorganisms into the lower airways from proximal sites, including the oral and nasal cavities.[1,2] This disease is particularly prevalent in, and problematic for, the elderly, especially those in institutions, such as nursing homes, and for those with several important risk factors. The role of the oral microbiota in this process—and the role of oral care in limiting it—is now well-recognized, because the bacteria that contribute to disease initiation often are aspirated from the oral cavity.

This article originally appeared in Dental Clinics, Volume 65 Issue 2, April 2021.
This article has been updated from *"Oral Health Disparities in Older Adults: Oral Bacteria, Inflammation, and Aspiration Pneumonia"* by Frank A. Scannapieco and Kenneth Shay, previously published in *Dental Clinics of North America*, Volume 58, Issue 4, October 2014.
Department of Oral Biology, School of Dental Medicine, University at Buffalo, The State University of New York, Foster Hall, 3435 Main Street, Buffalo, NY 14214, USA
E-mail address: fas1@buffalo.edu

Clin Geriatr Med 39 (2023) 257–271
https://doi.org/10.1016/j.cger.2023.01.010
0749-0690/23/© 2023 Elsevier Inc. All rights reserved.

Pneumonia is classified according to the location of the origin of the etiologic infectious agents (ie, from the community vs from within a health care institution, so called nosocomial pneumonia). One specific form of pneumonia, aspiration pneumonia (AP), is an infectious process caused by the aspiration of oropharyngeal secretions containing pathogenic bacteria.[2,3] This is differentiated from aspiration pneumonitis, which typically is caused by chemical injury following inhalation of sterile gastric contents. Although aspiration of small amounts of oropharyngeal secretions is normal in healthy persons during sleep, large-volume aspiration (macroaspiration) of oropharyngeal or upper gastrointestinal contents containing microorganisms drives the pathogenesis of AP, both in the community and in the health care delivery environment, such as the nursing home.[2] AP almost always is caused by a mixed infection, including oral bacteria (from the saliva and gingival crevice), and often develops in patients with elevated risk of aspiration of oral fluids into the lung, such as those with dysphagia or depressed consciousness.[1,4]

This article, which updates an article included in a previous volume on geriatric dentistry in *Dental Clinics of North America*,[5] reviews the epidemiology, microbiology, pathogenesis, and prevention of AP, with a focus on the role of poor oral health as a risk factor for, and dental care in the prevention and management of, this important infection.

EPIDEMIOLOGY

Together with influenza, pneumonia consistently ranks as the eighth most common cause of death in the United States.[6] In 2017, there were 55,672 cases of pneumonia/influenza in the United States. Among adults greater than or equal to 65 years of age, annual rates of hospitalized community-acquired pneumonia (CAP) ranged from 847 per 100,000 persons to 3500 per 100,000 persons, with a median of 1830 per 100,000 persons.[7]

Pneumonia is the second most common hospital-acquired pneumonia (HAP) in the United States (after urinary tract infection), representing 10% to 15% of these infections, and is associated with substantial morbidity, mortality, and cost.[8] Most patients who contract HAP are infants, young children, and persons greater than 65 years of age; persons with severe underlying disease, immunosuppression, or neurologic deficit; and patients undergoing abdominal surgery. Hospital-acquired infections are those that occur greater than 48 hours after admission to a hospital or other residential health care facility (such as a nursing home). Pneumonia is the most common infection in the intensive care unit (ICU) setting, accounting for 10% of infections in ICUs.[9] HAP can be divided further into 2 subtypes: ventilator-associated pneumonia (VAP) and non–ventilator-associated HAP.[10,11]

The classification scheme for pneumonia also considers that which occurs in health care delivery settings. For this reason, the term, *health care–associated pneumonia* (*HCAP*),[12] is used to describe the range of patients who could be affected. An important type of HCAP is nursing home–associated pneumonia (NHAP), the leading cause of death in the nursing home population.[13,14] The incidence of NHAP is estimated to range from 0.7 episode/1000 patient days to 1 episode/1000 patient days.[15] Mortality has been estimated to be 8% to 54%.[15] Pneumonia is the most common reason for transfer of nursing home residents to the hospital.[14] Because hospital-based treatment of NHAP is costly, practitioners often are compelled to provide treatment in the nursing home rather than after transfer of the patient to the hospital. There is evidence that there are no differences in outcomes when comparing NHAP treated by use of oral antibiotics in the nursing home versus parenteral treatment after hospitalization.[16]

Regarding AP, a retrospective study analyzed electronic medical records at a tertiary-care, university-affiliated hospital from 1996 to 2006 to understand the demographics of the disease.[17] Of 628 patients with AP, 510 cases were community acquired. The median age was 77 years, with 30-day mortality of 21%. Patients with community-acquired AP, compared with CAP patients, had more frequent inpatient admission (99% vs 58%, respectively) and ICU admission (38% vs 14%, respectively). These data demonstrate that patients with community-acquired AP are older, have more comorbidities, and demonstrate higher mortality than CAP patients.

The importance of pneumonia has been well illustrated as a result of the COVID-19 pandemic. It has been reported that angiotensin-converting enzyme 2 (ACE2) is the main host cell receptor of 2019 nVoV virus and plays a crucial role in the entry of the virus into the cell to cause the final infection. ACE2 is highly enriched in epithelial cells of tongue.[18] Thus, the oral cavity is a potential point of ingress for 2019-nCoV infection. Also, secondary bacterial infection is a potential serious sequelae of this disease,[19] and the oral cavity could be a source of bacteria aspirated into the lung. Future studies are needed to determine the role of the oral microbiota in this process. Such studies could reveal the potential for dental care and oral hygiene in prevention of secondary infection in COVID-19 and other patients with viral lung infections.

MICROBIOLOGY

It long has been thought that the lung is sterile, and the presence of any microbe in the lung is a sign of, and results in, infection.[20] This long-held assumption recently has been challenged by new studies using molecular techniques and sterile sampling approaches that have allowed for the assessment of microorganisms in all human tissues and organs. It now is appreciated that a complex microbial community resides on the surfaces of the lower airways of healthy subjects.[21] Until systems were devised to reliably obtain sterile samples from the lower airway, sputum often was the convenient sample of choice to investigate lung infections. It was assumed that bacteria from upper airway and the oral cavity found in sputum were contaminants and, therefore, not pertinent to the pathogenesis of lung infections. With the advent of the use of sterile bronchoalveolar lavage sampling techniques, it now is known that the lower airway in healthy subjects harbor small populations of bacteria in the lower airway. The evidence to date suggests that dispersal of microbes from the oral cavity is the primary driver of the healthy lung microbiome.[22] It is well known that AP patients often harbor multiple species of bacteria, often microbes normally indigenous to the oral cavity. Unfortunately, a comprehensive study of the microbiome of AP is not yet unavailable.

In mechanically ventilated patients, which involves placement of an endotracheal tube to provide oxygen into the lower airway, the tube often becomes colonized with microbes from the oral cavity, which subsequently forms a biofilm and promotes VAP. In ventilated patients, it has been shown that a microbial shift occurs in dental plaque, with colonization by potential VAP pathogens, which seed the lower airways via endotracheal tube biofilms.[23]

Several studies have used molecular approaches to characterize the microbiome of the lung with pneumonia.[24] For example, the microbiome of bronchoalveolar lavage fluid in Japanese patients with HAP found the most common bacteria identified were streptococci, *Corynebacterium* species, and anaerobes.[25] *Staphylococcus aureus*, *Klebsiella pneumoniae*, and *Escherichia coli* were found in patients with late-onset pneumonia. Another study used molecular techniques to assess the impact of oral hygiene status on the composition of the microbiome of the bronchoalveolar lavage fluid directly obtained from lungs suspected to have pneumonia. Poor oral hygiene was found significantly associated with anaerobes in the lungs of patients with pneumonia.[26]

Metataxonomics, a recently developed approach to assessing microbial diversity that uses data from high-throughput sequencing to identify microorganisms and viruses within a complex mixture, was used to simultaneously characterize the microbiome of dental plaque, endotracheal tubes, and nondirected bronchial lavages in mechanically ventilated patients to determine associations between these microbial communities.[27] No significant differences in the microbial communities between these samples were noted, and most bacteria detected were oral species and respiratory pathogens (S aureus, Pseudomonas aeruginosa, Streptococcus pneumoniae, and Haemophilus influenzae). These findings suggest that the oral cavity is a reservoir for the microbes that are aspirated into the lower airway and that attach to the endotracheal tube.

PATHOGENESIS

Under normal circumstances, the lower airway provides formidable defense against bacteria that are aspirated.[28] A viscous mucous layer coating the epithelium, containing host-derived mucins and antimicrobial components, such as lactoperoxidase, lysozyme, and other antimicrobial peptides,[29] traps most bacteria, which then are removed from the lung by the mucociliary escalator, the unidirectional beating of epithelial cilia that transports foreign mater and debris out of the lung. Complex bacterial surface components interact with mucosal cell pattern recognition receptors, such as Toll-like receptors, to activate inflammation through the nuclear factor κB signaling pathway. This in turn recruits activated macrophages and neutrophils that engulf the invading bacteria.

Pneumonia is the result of aspiration of infectious agents colonizing the oral cavity and/or upper respiratory tract.[30,31] Several mechanisms have been proposed to explain how microorganisms can enter the lung to cause infection. Any conditions that reduce containment of the secretions to the upper airway and that compromise upper airway defenses increase the risk for pneumonia by allowing aspirated bacteria to attach to the respiratory epithelium, which then triggers the cascade of events that result in overt infection (**Fig. 1**). It has been suggested that bacteria from the gastrointestinal tract may escape from the intestinal lumen into the mesenteric lymph nodes, then possibly to be transported systemically to the lung to cause pneumonia.[32] Clinical studies with critically ill patients, however, have not proved this route of infection to be the major cause of pneumonia. Another potential source of bacteria is the upper gastrointestinal tract, where bacteria could be regurgitated to the oropharynx and then aspirated.[33] Finally, colonization of the oral cavity by exogenous respiratory pathogens, or aspiration of the commensal bacteria that already colonize the teeth and oral tissue surfaces, can be aspirated to cause infection.[31]

Placement of an endotracheal tube through the larynx and trachea into the lung can provide a route for bacteria to bypass those structures that normally prevent aspiration, such as the glottis. Anything that diminishes salivary function and flow likely influences this process, including patients' use of pharmacologic agents that reduce salivary flow.[34,35]

Another important factor that promotes aspiration is dysphagia, which is more common in elderly individuals.[36] Dysphagia also is common in nursing home residents[37]

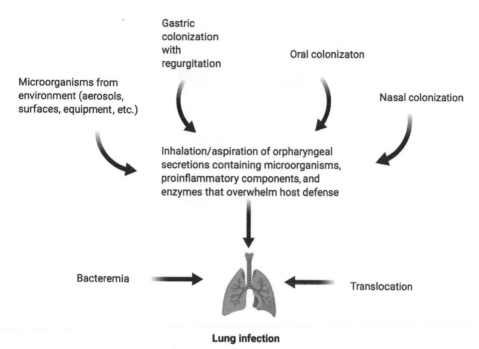

Fig. 1. Factors influencing pathogenesis of pneumonia.

and, therefore, represents an important risk factor for AP. It is possible that dysphagia can occur in the absence of overt signs of swallowing difficulty: so-called silent aspiration.[38] Certain conditions, such as stroke or impaired cough reflex, may increase the frequency of such silent aspiration.

It is likely that most cases of AP are the result of mixed infections involving 2 or more bacterial species, which may be more virulent than infections caused by a single species.[39] Disease can be initiated by bacteria normally indigenous to the oral cavity, especially anaerobes associated with periodontal disease.[40] Alternatively, these species may potentiate the pathogenic potential of other, more typical respiratory pathogens, such as *Streptococcus pneumonia*, *S aureus*, or *P aeruginosa*, which can colonize the oral cavity in high-risk subjects such as those in the nursing home.[41,42] It is well documented that potential respiratory pathogens, such as *S aureus*, *P aeruginosa*, *K pneumoniae*, and *Enterobacter cloacae*, colonize the dental plaque of dependent elderly.[43,44] In some health care settings, more than half the subjects assessed showed the presence of these bacteria in the dental plaque, and prevalence of colonization has been correlated with length of time in the setting.[4,31] The tongue also appears to be colonized by common respiratory pathogens, including *H influenzae*, *K pneumoniae*, *P aeruginosa*, *S aureus*, and *Streptococcus pneumoniae*.[45]

RISK FACTORS

Risk factors that have been associated with AP, along with a list of the major respiratory pathogens, are considered in **Fig. 2**. Dysphagia (swallowing dysfunction) likely is the most important risk factor for AP. Dysphagia is a relatively common finding in the elderly, the most common residents of nursing homes.[46] It is a result

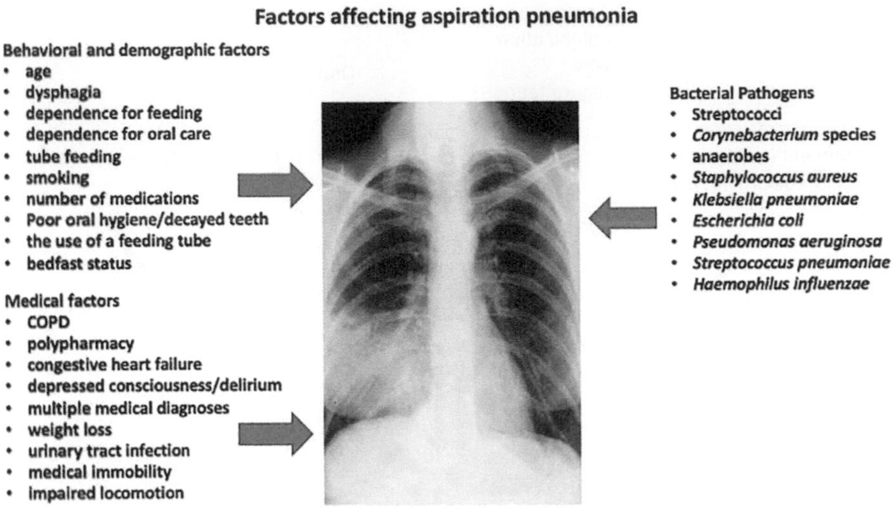

Factors affecting aspiration pneumonia

Behavioral and demographic factors
- age
- dysphagia
- dependence for feeding
- dependence for oral care
- tube feeding
- smoking
- number of medications
- Poor oral hygiene/decayed teeth
- the use of a feeding tube
- bedfast status

Medical factors
- COPD
- polypharmacy
- congestive heart failure
- depressed consciousness/delirium
- multiple medical diagnoses
- weight loss
- urinary tract infection
- medical immobility
- impaired locomotion

Bacterial Pathogens
- Streptococci
- *Corynebacterium* species
- anaerobes
- *Staphylococcus aureus*
- *Klebsiella pneumoniae*
- *Escherichia coli*
- *Pseudomonas aeruginosa*
- *Streptococcus pneumoniae*
- *Haemophilus influenzae*

Fig. 2. Risk factors and potential bacterial pathogens of AP.

of perturbation in the coordination of multiple muscle systems that control the functions of the oral cavity, pharynx and esophagus. Dysphagia often is associated with Parkinson disease, Alzheimer disease, stroke, other neurodegenerative condition, or advanced age.[47] A recent systematic review that sought to identify risk factors for AP found dysphagia to have the most robust positive correlation with AP (odds ratio 9.84; 95% CI, 4.15–23.33).[48] The significant predictors for AP from a prospective study of 189 elderly veterans residing in a Department of Veterans Affairs nursing home included dependence for feeding, dependence for oral care, tube feeding, currently smoking, multiple medical diagnoses, number of medications, and number of decayed teeth.[49] Another study that followed 358 institutionalized veterans aged 55 years and older found statistically significant risk factors for AP for patients with no natural teeth included chronic obstructive pulmonary disease (COPD), diabetes, dependence with feeding, and presence of *S aureus* in saliva.[50] Risk factors for patients with natural teeth included the preceding 4 plus number of decayed teeth, number of pairs of opposing teeth, and presence of decay-causing and periodontal disease—causing organisms in saliva or dental plaque.

A retrospective analysis of 3 states' Minimum Data Set/Resident Assessment Instrument reports for a 1-year period, representing approximately 100,000 nursing home residents, found the following risk indicators for AP: COPD, congestive heart failure, the use of a feeding tube, bedfast status, high case mix (low functionality/high dependency), delirium, weight loss, swallowing problems, urinary tract infection, mechanical diet, dependence for eating, medical immobility, impaired locomotion, number of medications, and age.[47]

More recently, modifiable risk factors for pneumonia in elderly nursing home residents were identified in a prospective study of 613 elderly residents of 5 nursing homes.[51] In this cohort, 18% developed pneumonia. Statistical modeling suggested that inadequate oral care and difficulty with swallowing were associated with pneumonia. Another comprehensive assessment of oral health using a revised oral assessment guide in older adults with pneumonia found a correlation between this score and aspiration risk.[52] Such a convenient tool might be useful to identify subjects with high risk to target preventive measures.

Thus, the drivers of AP are those that undermine swallowing function and oral hygiene as well as underlying medical conditions that reduce immune function. It, therefore, is no surprise that many elders are inherently at risk for AP.

ORAL HEALTH AND ASPIRATION PNEUMONIA

Prior to the mid-1990s, the role of oral conditions in the pathogenesis of AP, in particular, poor oral hygiene and periodontal inflammation, mostly was ignored in the medical and nursing care setting. This was in spite of the fact that it was understood that the source of many of the infectious agents causing the disease often was the oral microbiota. This situation began to change as knowledge of the specific role of the oral microflora in the pathogenesis of pneumonia became available.[1,31] Much of the work at this time was performed in hospitalized patients, in particular, mechanically ventilated patients in ICUs, who have substantially elevated risk for pneumonia. It was shown that the teeth serve as a reservoir for respiratory pathogen colonization[53–55] and thus serve as a source of bacteria in aspirated secretions. Further studies also suggested that methods to improve oral hygiene in these populations could reduce their risk of pneumonia.[56–61]

Several studies have shown that the oral cavity also might serve as a reservoir for pulmonary infection in nursing home residents.[43,44,62] Again, the oral cavities of elderly residents of nursing homes were found to harbor respiratory pathogens more frequently than those of ambulatory patients.

There also is some evidence that periodontal disease may be associated with risk for pneumonia in elderly patients. A study of an elderly Japanese population found that the adjusted mortality due to pneumonia was 3.9-times higher in persons with 10 or more teeth with a probing depth exceeding 4 mm (ie, with periodontal pockets) than in those without periodontal pockets.[63] A case-control study compared 85 cases with nosocomial pneumonia against 230 controls without nosocomial pneumonia, employing a full-mouth periodontal examination for all subjects.[64] Individuals with periodontitis had a 3-fold excess risk pneumonia compared with the control group without periodontal disease, following adjustment for a variety of potential confounding variables. It also has been suggested that the number of teeth also may have an impact on risk for pneumonia, with a direct relationship between number of teeth lost and pneumonia reported.[65]

In light of these findings, it seems intuitively obvious that oral hygiene or periodontal therapy help prevent the onset or progression of AP in high-risk patients. Several studies, discussed later, have tested this hypothesis. Several studies have evaluated the effectiveness of oral care to prevent pneumonia in nursing home patients, for example, mechanical oral care, in some cases in combination with povidone iodine, was shown to have a moderate effect in reducing the risk of pneumonia in nursing home residents.[66–69] A recent study that the loss of oral self-care ability along with gender (male) and malnutrition has been shown to increase the risk for pneumonia in elderly patients.[70] In addition, once-a-week professional oral cleaning significantly reduced influenza infections in an elderly population.[71]

Implementation of professional oral care programs in nursing facilities, involving the deployment of dental hygienists to provide direct oral care, including tooth, tongue, and denture brushing, may help reduce the oropharyngeal microbial burden and, therefore, the number of microbes that can be aspirated into the lower airway.[72] Such an approach also may reduce the risk of other respiratory infections, such as influenza.[73] This idea is supported by a recent systematic review of reported evidence that oral care interventions given by dental personnel were more effective than oral care interventions given by nurses on mortality from HCAP in elderly adults in hospitals.[74]

Some studies have not supported the effectiveness of oral care to prevent pneumonia in the nursing home.[75] A unique cluster-randomized study of 834 nursing home patients, followed over the course of a year, showed no benefit of a comprehensive oral care program, which included tooth brushing, topical chlorhexidine, and upright positioning during feeding. The lack of effect could be explained by several possibilities, including less than ideal staff adherence to the intervention protocol, control usual oral care group may have been modified after study initiation to more closely resemble the intervention arm, and changes in the microbial flora over time in response to the implementation of the intervention.

Overall, oral cleansing protocols have been shown to reduce pneumonia in both edentulous and dentate subjects, suggesting that oral colonization of bacteria contributes to nosocomial pneumonia to a greater extent than periodontitis per se. However, intervention studies where periodontitis is treated and the incidence of pneumonia is then measured have not been performed due to the complexities imposed by ICU or bedbound nursing home patients. It has been suggested that dental services are underutilized by nursing home residents. Thus, more effort must be made to improve the frequency and effectiveness of oral care protocols on nursing homes.[76]

In edentulous patients, dentures conceivably could serve as a reservoir for oral and respiratory bacterial colonization similar to teeth if not cleaned properly on a daily basis, although neither removable dentures nor the edentulous oral cavity provides the anaerobic environments favored by periodontopathic organisms. Recent studies suggest that putative respiratory pathogens (S aureus, Streptococcus pneumoniae, P aeruginosa, H influenzae type b, Streptococcus pyogenes, and Moraxella catarrhalis) colonize a majority of dentures.[77] Daily cleaning of dentures may help prevent pneumonia.[78] A recent study found that that elders who wear dentures during sleep double their risk for pneumonia.[79] This finding underscores the potential role for dentures in pneumonia risk.

At the population level, frequent periodontal care may reduce the risk for pneumonia. A recent study investigated the association between periodontal treatment and the risk of pneumonia events in a Taiwanese cohort assembled from the Taiwanese National Health Insurance Research Database. Results suggest that patients having periodontal treatment exhibited a significantly lower risk of pneumonia than the general population.[80]

SUGGESTIONS FOR ORAL CARE OF DEPENDENT, ELDERLY PATIENTS TO PREVENT ASPIRATION PNEUMONIA

Review of the literature reveals several actions to take that could reduce the risk of AP in high-risk patients. Numerous studies have linked aspiration of microorganisms from dental plaque with risk for pneumonia. Although the evidence is strongest in cases of VAP and NHAP, there is no reason to believe this does not apply in the case of patients at high risk for AP. Several studies have demonstrated that improved oral hygiene can reduce the risk of pneumonia in nursing home residents.[81] More recently, modifiable risk factors for pneumonia in elderly nursing home residents were identified in a prospective study of 613 elderly residents of 5 nursing homes.[51] In this cohort, 18% developed pneumonia. Statistical modeling suggested that inadequate oral care and difficulty with swallowing were associated with pneumonia. Another comprehensive assessment of oral health using a revised oral assessment guide in older adults with pneumonia found a correlation between this score and aspiration risk.[52] Such a convenient tool might be useful to identify subjects with high risk to target preventive measures.

Residents of ICUs arguably are generally less able than nursing home residents to attend to their own daily care needs, due to the extent of infirmity, altered consciousness, and the presence of physical impediments (eg, ventilator, feeding, and intravenous tubes; restraints). But individuals are placed in nursing home settings because 1 or more of their essential daily care needs, such as bathing, dressing, transferring, toileting, and eating, cannot be adequately addressed without the services provided in such a facility.[82] For example, the 2010 National Nursing Home Survey reported that more than 72% of the approximately 1.5 million Americans residing in nursing homes are dependent on the assistance of another for addressing their bathing needs (including oral and hair care). And, in contrast to ICU settings, where lengths of stay vary from days to weeks, length of stay in nursing home generally is counted in weeks, months, or years. Unmet daily oral care that is not addressed on behalf of a nursing home resident is likely, over time, to pose a greater threat than the same need in an ICU patient.

Numerous studies have reported on the high prevalence of very poor oral conditions, including inadequate provision of daily oral hygiene, observed in both dentate and edentulous residents of nursing homes.[83,84] The situation is underscored by a recent study that described factors associated with the utilization of dental services in.[76] The records of 2516 residents discharged from a long-term care facility in a nursing home. Western New York between 2008 and 2012 were evaluated to document utilization of dental services. The author found that only 10.3% of residents utilized dental services at least once during their stay. Those who utilized dental services, compared with those who did not utilize dental services, were significantly older at admission (78.5 y vs 82.0 years, respectively; $P<.001$), stayed longer (1.6 y vs 3.9 y, respectively; $P<.001$), were more likely to be female (63.6% vs 75.6%, respectively; $P = .008$), and were less likely to be married (37.7% vs 14.0%, respectively; $P \leq.001$). Thus, at least in some cases, dental services appear to be underutilized by residents of long-term care facilities.

Several factors may contribute to the under-provision of oral care in long-term care settings.[85–88] The recommended staffing ratio of nurse:patients often is low in a nursing home, limiting the staff time available for delivering needed care. Although ICUs are staffed by registered nurses, nurse aides deliver most care in nursing homes. Studies have demonstrated strong correlations among nursing home staff between duration of nurse training, patiant income and the importance accorded to personal health as well as patient's oral health. Oral anatomy, oral assessment, and provision of daily oral care are seldom part of nursing curricula, emphasizing the importance of in-service education and establishing and following protocols, such as the ICU bundles, described previously. Nurse aides in long-term care have the highest annual turnover of any clinical position, undermining any potential impact of educational interventions directed at enhancing performance. Finally, the dominant payment sources for ICU services (eg, Medicare and insurance) ultimately must bear the cost of AP, which compels clinical managers to seek out and adopt practices that can prevent onset of the disease. In contrast, the dominant payment source for nursing home care (Medicaid) will not bear the cost for hospitalization due to AP or even pneumonia care undertaken within the nursing home (Medicare), limiting the impetus for undertaking AP-prevention measures.

CLINICS CARE POINTS

Based on the information in this article, several recommendations can be considered for prevention of AP in frail elderly residents of nursing homes. These include

- Oral hygiene conducted several times a day using a soft bristled toothbrush, fluoridated dentifrice for 3 minutes to 4 minutes, and dental floss (if possible) to remove debris and dental plaque at least twice a day
- The use of an antibacterial oral rinse
- Regular tooth cleaning by a dentist or hygienists, as needed
- Daily denture hygiene using a denture brush; removal of oral appliances, such as full or partial dentures while sleeping

SUMMARY

Most factors that influence the pathogenesis of AP affect swallowing function, oral hygiene, or host susceptibility and underlying medical conditions. It should come as no surprise that many elders, therefore, are inherently at risk for AP. The importance of oral care for elders to prevent AP cannot be overemphasized. Oral preventive measures can reduce the risk for AP, especially for hospitalized, institutionalized, and disabled elderly. Reduction of oral biofilm in these populations reduces the numbers of potential respiratory pathogens in the oral secretions that can be aspirated, which, in turn, reduces the risk for pneumonia. Effective oral hygiene, together with other preventive measures (correct head-of-bed position for bedbound patients; promotion of salivary flow; vaccination against known respiratory pathogens, such as *Streptococcus pneumoniae;* management of swallowing disorders; proper daily denture care; and so forth), helps control lower respiratory infections in vulnerable patients. Unfortunately, oral hygiene practice resulting in complete removal of oral biofilms from teeth and other oral surfaces is difficult to accomplish. Adoption of stringent oral hygiene practice in these patients may become more widespread if additional actions are taken. Conduct of large-scale clinical trials to test novel oral care interventions are tested. Enhancing educational activities to improve knowledge of oral care procedures for caregivers (eg, for nurses and family care givers) would have an important impact. Further studies of the basic microbiology of AP, as well as antimicrobial strategies targeting appropriate members of the lung microbiota, will help inform clinicians and researchers who design trials. Finally, funding agencies would be wise to consider support of research addressing this issue that could pay off in preventing a large number of cases and reduce the morbidity and cost of treating this dreadful disease.

DISCLOSURE

The author has nothing to disclose.

REFERENCES

1. Raghavendran K, Mylotte JM, Scannapieco FA. Nursing home-associated pneumonia, hospital-acquired pneumonia and ventilator-associated pneumonia: the contribution of dental biofilms and periodontal inflammation. Periodontol 2000 2007;44:164–77.
2. Mandell LA, Niederman MS. Aspiration pneumonia. N Engl J Med 2019;380(7): 651–63.

3. Marik PE. Aspiration pneumonitis and aspiration pneumonia. N Engl J Med 2001; 344(9):665–71.
4. Shay K, Scannapieco FA, Terpenning MS, et al. Nosocomial pneumonia and oral health. Spec Care Dentist 2005;25(4):179–87.
5. Scannapieco FA, Shay K. Oral health disparities in older adults: oral bacteria, inflammation, and aspiration pneumonia. Dent Clin North Am 2014;58(4):771–82.
6. Kochanek KD, Murphy SL, Xu JQ, et al. Deaths: final data for 2017. National Center for Health Statistics; 2019.
7. McLaughlin JM, Khan FL, Thoburn EA, et al. Rates of hospitalization for community-acquired pneumonia among US adults: a systematic review. Vaccine 2020;38(4):741–51.
8. Flanders SA, Collard HR, Saint S. Nosocomial pneumonia: state of the science. Am J Infect Control 2006;34(2):84–93.
9. Vincent JL, Bihari DJ, Suter PM, et al. The prevalence of nosocomial infection in intensive care units in Europe. Results of the European prevalence of infection in intensive care (EPIC) Study. EPIC international advisory committee. JAMA 1995; 274(8):639–44.
10. Giuliano KK, Baker D, Quinn B. The epidemiology of nonventilator hospital-acquired pneumonia in the United States. Am J Infect Control 2018;46(3):322–7.
11. Baker D, Quinn B. Hospital acquired pneumonia prevention initiative-2: incidence of nonventilator hospital-acquired pneumonia in the United States. Am J Infect Control 2018;46(1):2–7.
12. Tablan OC, Anderson LJ, Besser R, et al. Guidelines for preventing health-care–associated pneumonia, 2003: recommendations of CDC and the healthcare infection control practices advisory committee. MMWR Recomm Rep 2004; 53(RR-3):1–36.
13. Mylotte JM. Nursing home-acquired pneumonia. Clin Infect Dis 2002;35(10): 1205–11.
14. Muder RR. Pneumonia in residents of long-term care facilities: epidemiology, etiology, management, and prevention. Am J Med 1998;105(4):319–30.
15. Mylotte JM. Nursing home-associated pneumonia. Clin Geriatr Med 2007;23(3): 553–65, vi-vii.
16. Dosa D. Should I hospitalize my resident with nursing home-acquired pneumonia? J Am Med Dir Assoc 2006;7(3 Suppl):S74–80, 73.
17. Lanspa MJ, Jones BE, Brown SM, et al. Mortality, morbidity, and disease severity of patients with aspiration pneumonia. J Hosp Med 2013;8(2):83–90.
18. Xu H, Zhong L, Deng J, et al. High expression of ACE2 receptor of 2019-nCoV on the epithelial cells of oral mucosa. Int J Oral Sci 2020;12(1):8.
19. Li X, Wang L, Yan S, et al. Clinical characteristics of 25 death cases with COVID-19: a retrospective review of medical records in a single medical center, Wuhan, China. Int J Infect Dis 2020;94:128–32.
20. Donowitz GR, Mandell GL. Acute pneumonia. In: Mandell GL, Douglas RG, Bennett JE, editors. Principles and practice of infectious diseases. New York (NY): Churchill Liningstone; 1990. p. 540–55.
21. Segal LN, Rom WN, Weiden MD. Lung microbiome for clinicians. New discoveries about bugs in healthy and diseased lungs. Ann Am Thorac Soc 2014; 11(1):108–16.
22. Venkataraman A, Bassis CM, Beck JM, et al. Application of a neutral community model to assess structuring of the human lung microbiome. mBio 2015;6(1): e02284-14.

23. Sands KM, Wilson MJ, Lewis MAO, et al. Respiratory pathogen colonization of dental plaque, the lower airways, and endotracheal tube biofilms during mechanical ventilation. J Crit Care 2017;37:30–7.

24. Yin Y, Hountras P, Wunderink RG. The microbiome in mechanically ventilated patients. Curr Opin Infect Dis 2017;30(2):208–13.

25. Yatera K, Noguchi S, Yamasaki K, et al. Determining the possible etiology of hospital-acquired pneumonia using a clone library analysis in Japan. Tohoku J Exp Med 2017;242(1):9–17.

26. Hata R, Noguchi S, Kawanami T, et al. Poor oral hygiene is associated with the detection of obligate anaerobes in pneumonia. J Periodontol 2020;91(1):65–73.

27. Marino PJ, Wise MP, Smith A, et al. Community analysis of dental plaque and endotracheal tube biofilms from mechanically ventilated patients. J Crit Care 2017;39:149–55.

28. Gellatly SL, Hancock RE. Pseudomonas aeruginosa: new insights into pathogenesis and host defenses. Pathog Dis 2013;67(3):159–73.

29. Gerson C, Sabater J, Scuri M, et al. The lactoperoxidase system functions in bacterial clearance of airways. Am J Respir Cell Mol Biol 2000;22(6):665–71.

30. Johanson WG, Dever LL. Nosocomial pneumonia. Intensive Care Med 2003; 29(1):23–9.

31. Scannapieco FA. Role of oral bacteria in respiratory infection. J Periodontol 1999; 70(7):793–802.

32. Assimakopoulos SF, Triantos C, Thomopoulos K, et al. Gut-origin sepsis in the critically ill patient: pathophysiology and treatment. Infection 2018;46(6):751–60.

33. Estes RJ, GU Meduri. The pathogenesis of ventilator-associated pneumonia: mechanisms of bacterial translocation and airway inoculation. Intensive Care Med 1995;21:365–83.

34. Gibson G, Barrett E. The role of salivary function on oropharyngeal colonization. Spec Care Dentist 1992;12(4):153–6.

35. Gupta A, Epstein JB, Sroussi H. Hyposalivation in elderly patients. J Can Dent Assoc 2006;72(9):841–6.

36. Sue Eisenstadt E. Dysphagia and aspiration pneumonia in older adults. J Am Acad Nurse Pract 2010;22(1):17–22.

37. Park YH, Han HR, Oh BM, et al. Prevalence and associated factors of dysphagia in nursing home residents. Geriatr Nurs 2013;34(3):212–7.

38. Ramsey D, Smithard D, Kalra L. Silent aspiration: what do we know? Dysphagia 2005;20(3):218–25.

39. Kimizuka R, Kato T, Ishihara K, et al. Mixed infections with Porphyromonas gingivalis and Treponema denticola cause excessive inflammatory responses in a mouse pneumonia model compared with monoinfections. Microbes Infect 2003;5(15):1357–62.

40. Bartlett JG. Anaerobic bacterial infection of the lung. Anaerobe 2012;18(2): 235–9.

41. Pan Y, Teng D, Burke AC, et al. Oral bacteria modulate invasion and induction of apoptosis in HEp-2 cells by Pseudomonas aeruginosa. Microb Pathog 2009; 46(2):73–9.

42. Li X, Guo H, Tian Q, et al. Effects of 5-aminolevulinic acid-mediated photodynamic therapy on antibiotic-resistant staphylococcal biofilm: an in vitro study. J Surg Res 2013;184(2):1013–21.

43. Russell SL, Boylan RJ, Kaslick RS, et al. Respiratory pathogen colonization of the dental plaque of institutionalized elders. Spec Care Dentist 1999;19:1–7.

44. Sumi Y, Miura H, Michiwaki Y, et al. Colonization of dental plaque by respiratory pathogens in dependent elderly. Arch Gerontol Geriatr 2007;44(2):119–24.
45. Hong C, Aung MM, Kanagasabai K, et al. The association between oral health status and respiratory pathogen colonization with pneumonia risk in institutionalized adults. Int J Dent Hyg 2018;16(2):e96–102.
46. Marik PE, Kaplan D. Aspiration pneumonia and dysphagia in the elderly. Chest 2003;124(1):328–36.
47. Langmore SE, Skarupski KA, Park PS, et al. Predictors of aspiration pneumonia in nursing home residents. Dysphagia 2002;17(4):298–307.
48. van der Maarel-Wierink CD, Vanobbergen JN, Bronkhorst EM, et al. Meta-analysis of dysphagia and aspiration pneumonia in frail elders. J Dent Res 2011; 90(12):1398–404.
49. Langmore SE, Terpenning MS, Schork A, et al. Predictors of aspiration pneumonia: how important is dysphagia? Dysphagia 1998;13:69–81.
50. Terpenning MS, Taylor GW, Lopatin DE, et al. Aspiration pneumonia: dental and oral risk factors in an older veteran population. J Am Geriatr Soc 2001;49:557–63.
51. Quagliarello V, Ginter S, Han L, et al. Modifiable risk factors for nursing home-acquired pneumonia. Clin Infect Dis 2005;40(1):1–6.
52. Noguchi S, Yatera K, Kato T, et al. Using oral health assessment to predict aspiration pneumonia in older adults. Gerodontology 2018;35(2):110–6.
53. Scannapieco FA, Stewart EM, Mylotte JM. Colonization of dental plaque by respiratory pathogens in medical intensive care patients. Crit Care Med 1992; 20(6):740–5.
54. El-Solh AA, Pietrantoni C, Bhat A, et al. Colonization of dental plaques: a reservoir of respiratory pathogens for hospital-acquired pneumonia in institutionalized elders. Chest 2004;126(5):1575–82.
55. Heo SM, Haase EM, Lesse AJ, et al. Genetic relationships between respiratory pathogens isolated from dental plaque and bronchoalveolar lavage fluid from patients in the intensive care unit undergoing mechanical ventilation. Clin Infect Dis 2008;47(12):1562–70.
56. Scannapieco FA, Bush RB, Paju S. Associations between periodontal disease and risk for nosocomial bacterial pneumonia and chronic obstructive pulmonary disease. A systematic review. Ann Periodontol 2003;8(1):54–69.
57. Azarpazhooh A, Leake JL. Systematic review of the association between respiratory diseases and oral health. J Periodontol 2006;77(9):1465–82.
58. Chan EY, Ruest A, Meade MO, et al. Oral decontamination for prevention of pneumonia in mechanically ventilated adults: systematic review and meta-analysis. BMJ 2007;334(7599):889.
59. Labeau SO, Van de Vyver K, Brusselaers N, et al. Prevention of ventilator-associated pneumonia with oral antiseptics: a systematic review and meta-analysis. Lancet Infect Dis 2011;11(11):845–54.
60. Roberts N, Moule P. Chlorhexidine and tooth-brushing as prevention strategies in reducing ventilator-associated pneumonia rates. Nurs Crit Care 2011;16(6): 295–302.
61. Shi Z, Xie H, Wang P, et al. Oral hygiene care for critically ill patients to prevent ventilator-associated pneumonia. Cochrane Database Syst Rev 2013;8: CD008367.
62. Didilescu AC, Skaug N, Marica C, et al. Respiratory pathogens in dental plaque of hospitalized patients with chronic lung diseases. Clin Oral Investig 2005;9(3): 141–7.

63. Awano S, Ansai T, Takata Y, et al. Oral health and mortality risk from pneumonia in the elderly. J Dent Res 2008;87(4):334–9.
64. Gomes-Filho IS, de Oliveira TF, da Cruz SS, et al. Influence of periodontitis in the development of nosocomial pneumonia: a case control study. J Periodontol 2014; 85(5):e82–90.
65. Suma S, Naito M, Wakai K, et al. Tooth loss and pneumonia mortality: a cohort study of Japanese dentists. PLoS One 2018;13(4):e0195813.
66. Adachi M, Ishihara K, Abe S, et al. Effect of professional oral health care on the elderly living in nursing homes. Oral Surg Oral Med Oral Pathol Oral Radiol Endod 2002;94(2):191–5.
67. Yoneyama T, Hashimoto K, Fukuda H, et al. Oral hygiene reduces respiratory infections in elderly bed-bound nursing home patients. Arch Gerontol Geriatr 1996; 22:11–9.
68. Yoneyama T, Yoshida M, Ohrui T, et al. Oral care reduces pneumonia in older patients in nursing homes. J Am Geriatr Soc 2002;50(3):430–3.
69. Liu C, Cao Y, Lin J, et al. Oral care measures for preventing nursing home-acquired pneumonia. Cochrane Database Syst Rev 2018;9:CD012416.
70. Fujiwara A, Minakuchi H, Uehara J, et al. Loss of oral self-care ability results in a higher risk of pneumonia in older inpatients: A prospective cohort study in a Japanese rural hospital. Gerodontology 2019;36(3):236–43.
71. Molloy J, Wolff LF, Lopez-Guzman A, et al. The association of periodontal disease parameters with systemic medical conditions and tobacco use. J Clin Periodontol 2004;31(8):625–32.
72. Ishikawa A, Yoneyama T, Hirota K, et al. Professional oral health care reduces the number of oropharyngeal bacteria. J Dent Res 2008;87(6):594–8.
73. Abe S, Ishihara K, Adachi M, et al. Oral hygiene evaluation for effective oral care in preventing pneumonia in dentate elderly. Arch Gerontol Geriatr 2005;43(1): 53–64.
74. Sjogren P, Wardh I, Zimmerman M, et al. Oral care and mortality in older adults with pneumonia in hospitals or nursing homes: systematic review and meta-analysis. J Am Geriatr Soc 2016;64(10):2109–15.
75. Juthani-Mehta M, Van Ness PH, McGloin J, et al. A cluster-randomized controlled trial of a multicomponent intervention protocol for pneumonia prevention among nursing home elders. Clin Infect Dis 2015;60(6):849–57.
76. Scannapieco FA, Amin S, Salme M, et al. Factors associated with utilization of dental services in a long-term care facility: a descriptive cross-sectional study. Spec Care Dentist 2017;37(2):78–84.
77. O'Donnell LE, Smith K, Williams C, et al. Dentures are a reservoir for respiratory pathogens. J Prosthodont 2015;25(2):99–104.
78. Kusama T, Aida J, Yamamoto T, et al. Infrequent denture cleaning increased the risk of pneumonia among community-dwelling older adults: a population-based cross-sectional study. Sci Rep 2019;9(1):13734.
79. Iinuma T, Arai Y, Abe Y, et al. Denture wearing during sleep doubles the risk of pneumonia in the very elderly. J Dent Res 2015;94(3 Suppl):28S–36S.
80. Yang LC, Suen YJ, Wang YH, et al. The association of periodontal treatment and decreased pneumonia: a nationwide population-based cohort study. Int J Environ Res Public Health 2020;17(1).
81. Sjogren P, Nilsson E, Forsell M, et al. A systematic review of the preventive effect of oral hygiene on pneumonia and respiratory tract infection in elderly people in hospitals and nursing homes: effect estimates and methodological quality of randomized controlled trials. J Am Geriatr Soc 2008;56(11):2124–30.

82. Katz TF, Walke LM, Suri R, et al. Goals of care for hospitalized nursing home residents. J Am Geriatr Soc 2001;49(6):837–8.
83. Berkey DB, Berg RG, Ettinger DL, et al. Research review of oral health status and service use among institutionalized older adults in the United States and Canada. Spec Care Dentist 1991;11:131–6.
84. Kiyak HA, Grayston MN, Crinean CL. Oral health problems and needs of nursing home residents. Community Dent Oral Epidemiol 1993;21:49–52.
85. Chalmers JM, Levy SM, Buckwalter KC, et al. Factors influencing nurses' aides' provision of oral care for nursing facility residents. Spec Care Dentist 1996; 16(2):71–9.
86. Wardh I, Andersson L, Sorensen S. Staff attitudes to oral health care. A comparative study of registered nurses, nursing assistants and home care aides. Gerodontology 1997;14(1):28–32.
87. Frenkel HF. Behind the screens: care staff observations on delivery of oral health care in nursing homes. Gerodontology 1999;16(2):75–80.
88. Chung JP, Mojon P, Budtz-Jorgensen E. Dental care of elderly in nursing homes: perceptions of managers, nurses, and physicians. Spec Care Dentist 2000; 20(1):12–7.

Oral Implications of Polypharmacy in Older Adults

Annetty P. Soto, DMD[a],*, Sarah L. Meyer, MLIS[b]

KEYWORDS

- Polypharmacy • Aged • Oral manifestations • Xerostomia
- Medication reconciliation

KEY POINTS

- Aged populations are at risk for polypharmacy.
- Medications have adverse side effects with oral manifestations.
- Diagnosis, treatment, and management of oral lesions are essential.
- Medication reconciliation should be integrated.

INTRODUCTION

Global demographics are being transformed by rapid acceleration of populations aged 65 and older and increasing life expectancy.[1] For instance, over one decade (2010–2019) in the United States the size of the 65-and-older population increased by one-third, the fastest growth of any age group.[2] The magnitude of this growth varies by state and ranges from 11% to 21% of the national population.[2] The US Census Bureau estimates by 2034 for the first time in the nation's history those 65 and older will outnumber children.[3] Simultaneously, life expectancy is increasing worldwide, but this trend is not associated with healthier populations.[1] The World Health Organization reports a contributor to a negative association between extended life expectancy and lack of health is multimorbidity, the presence of more than 1 chronic condition, which is elevated in aged populations.[4] The cumulative effect of chronic conditions on multiple body systems places aged populations at increased risk for common clinical geriatric syndromes, such as falls, frailty, cognitive decline, delirium, incontinence, and polypharmacy.[5]

This article originally appeared in Dental Clinics, Volume 65 Issue 2, April 2021.
[a] Division of General Dentistry, Department of Restorative Dental Sciences, University of Florida College of Dentistry, 1395 Center Drive, PO Box 100415, Gainesville, FL 32610-0415, USA; [b] University of Florida Health Science Center Libraries, 1600 Southwest Archer Road, PO Box 100206, Gainesville, FL 32610, USA
* Corresponding author.
E-mail address: asoto@dental.ufl.edu

Clin Geriatr Med 39 (2023) 273–293
https://doi.org/10.1016/j.cger.2023.01.008
0749-0690/23/Published by Elsevier Inc.

geriatric.theclinics.com

Most efforts to define the phenomenon of polypharmacy have primarily focused on a numerical threshold of coprescribed medications as a required criterion. Results of a recent review confirmed 46.6% of studies selected defined polypharmacy primarily in terms of a numerical threshold of coprescribing 5 or more medications. A small minority, 6% of studies, described an evolving concept focused on distinctions between inappropriate and appropriate polypharmacy.[6] Other researchers have sought to gauge appropriateness of polypharmacy.[7] A challenge of evaluating the appropriateness of polypharmacy is that multiple drugs are often prescribed with inadequate clinical indications or a lack of evidence base as an effective, safe, treatment strategy. Subsequently, patients potentially receive inappropriate polypharmacy and take prescriptions for extended periods and/or at excessive doses.[8]

Prevalence

Some experts believe that prevalence of multimorbidities is a driver of polypharmacy rates for older adults. In 2012, for Americans aged 65 or older, 61% had 2 or more chronic conditions.[9] Surveys in 2016 confirmed 41% of Americans, aged 65 or older was prescribed 5 or more drugs in the past 30 days.[10] Forty percent of community-dwelling and 75% of institutionalized older adults are concurrently prescribed 5 or more medications, whereas approximately 10% of older adults are prescribed 10 or more.[11]

Nature of the problem

Risks and challenges of polypharmacy are listed in **Box 1**.

Box 1
Risks and challenges of polypharmacy

Adverse drug reactions[a]

Potentially inappropriate prescriptions[a]

Medication nonadherence[a]

Drug duplication[a]

Drug-drug interactions[a]

Higher health care costs[a]

Morbidity and mortality[a]

Complexities associated with multimorbidities and polypharmacy increase the risk of fatal adverse drug events in aged populations (currently one of the 10 most common causes of death).[b]

Older patients are predisposed to adverse drug reactions because of consumption of large quantities of drugs and because of age-related changes in metabolism and patterns of drug usage.[c]

For all health care providers, presence of multimorbidities increases the challenges of assessing the safety and appropriateness of polypharmacy.

Other challenges in delivery and assessment of appropriate polypharmacy include lack of provider-provider care coordination, segregation of medical and dental care, limited clinician time to review and assess adverse reaction profiles of multiple drugs, and limitations in drug information resources to evaluate multiple drug-drug interactions.[d]

[a] Data from World Health Organization,[4] Michocki.[8] [b] Data from Quinn and Shah.[9] [c] Data from German and Burton.[12] [d] Data from Atchinson et al,[13] Nam et al,[14] Komiya et al,[15] Duke et al.[16]

Clinical Relevance

Increases in aged populations ensure that oral health providers will more frequently encounter patients with age-related physiologic changes in the oral cavity caused by comorbidities of chronic illnesses and changes resulting from medications used to manage diseases.[15] Therefore, it is essential to be trained to recognize risk factors of polypharmacy, diagnose, and treat oral lesions related to oral manifestations of clinical pharmacology and potential adversities to ensure delivery of safe and effective dental care.[17]

DISCUSSION

The 2000 Surgeon General's Report on Oral Health involved understanding of oral health and described its essential role in systemic health and well-being.[18] This report also highlighted the concept of the oral cavity as the "window" to the body and the importance of the oral-systematic connection. This connection is evident with estimates that more than one hundred systematic conditions and nearly five hundred medications exhibit oral manifestations.[19]

With increases in systemic diseases, comorbidities, and life expectancy, oral health care providers will have to be knowledgeable and ready to apply principles of geriatric medicine for the provision of care. Polypharmacy is one of the most common geriatric disorders (**Table 1**).

Oral Manifestations of Polypharmacy (Multiple Medications)

The indication for prescribed medications must be balanced against the potential for adverse effects. Drug-induced cutaneous reactions are common and varied in presentation, but only a limited number of reaction patterns occur in the oral cavity.[23] The most common medication-induced oral manifestations are detailed in this review and summarized in **Box 2**.

Aphthous-Like and Non-Aphthous-like Ulcers

"Aphthous-like" ulcers are oral ulcers whereby there is a known cause, resolving when the underlying cause is effectively managed.[23] This type of ulcer has a multifactorial

Table 1
Most prevalent risk factors for polypharmacy in older patients

Several chronic medical conditions	Attempts to direct how/what is prescribed
Aged 75 or older	Frailty
Deficient care coordination	Use of over-the-counter medications and/or herbal supplements
Frequent hospitalizations and/emergency room visits	Lack of caregivers
Nursing home placement	Multiple physicians from different specialties
Cognitive impairment	Socioeconomic factors (access to consistent care, inability to afford medications)
Use of additional substances (nonprescribed) to manage drug-induced condition	

Data from Refs.[20–22]

Box 2
Most common medication-induced oral manifestations

- Aphthous-like and non-aphthous-like ulcers
- Angioedema
- Dysesthesias (alteration in taste and burning mouth syndrome)
- Fungal and viral infections
- Fibrovascular hyperplasia
- Lichenoid reaction/lichen planus
- Xerostomia/salivary hyposalivation (caries risk, dysphagia)

Data from Halpern LR. The Geriatric Syndrome and Oral Health: Navigating Oral Disease Treatment Strategies in the Elderly. Dent Clin North Am. Jan 2020;64(1):209-228; and Yuan A, Woo SB. Adverse drug events in the oral cavity. Oral Surg Oral Med Oral Pathol Oral Radiol. Jan 2015;119(1):35-47.

---

cause and is frequently observed when dry mouth is associated with loss of lubrication and resultant trauma. Many case reports document that exposure to certain medications produces aphthous lesions as well.[24] Medications, including nonsteroidal anti-inflammatory drugs, antibiotics, β-blockers, angiotensin-converting enzyme (ACE) inhibitors, and antianginal medications, have all been implicated with oral ulceration lesions.[25]

A multivariate paired analysis revealed a significant association between nonsteroidal anti-inflammatory agents combined with β-blocker use and aphthous stomatitis.[26] Drug-induced ulcers are located on the side of the tongue, are solitary, and are resistant to usual treatments until the suspect medication is discontinued.[27] Nicorandil, prescribed to manage coronary artery disease, is linked to recurrent oral ulceration.[28] It is also associated with a deferred appearance of oral and gastrointestinal ulcers, and delayed appearance can take as long as 74 weeks to develop, with patients on high-dose regimens presenting sooner (**Fig. 1**).

Observational data and case studies report that many other drugs are associated with aphthous ulceration and stomatitis, including gold salts used for rheumatoid arthritis, and some selective serotonin reuptake inhibitors used for depression, ACE inhibitors, and drugs that affect the immune system, including interferons[29] (**Table 2**).

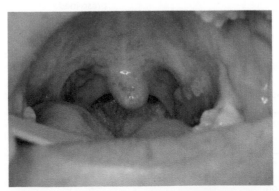

Fig. 1. Aphthous-like ulcer. (*Courtesy of* Dr. Mohammed Nadimul Islam, D.D.S., B.D.S, Florida.)

Table 2 Management strategies: aphthous-like and non-aphthous-like ulcers	
Clinical presentation	• Majority <1 cm, resolve in 5–14 d without scarring • Less than 10%, >1 cm, and scar[a]
Risk factors considerations	• Tobacco cessation (decreased recurrences)
Topical treatment recommendations	• Anesthetics • Lidocaine 1% cream, 2% gel, or spray[b] • Polidocanol paste • Benzocaine lozenges[b] • Chlorhexidine mouthwash and chamomile extract (improve healing, reduce frequency and severity)[a] • Chlortetracycline 2.5% mouthwash (improved ulcer and pain-free days by 40% compared with placebo)[c]
Therapeutic options for pain management	• Diclofenac 3% in 2.5% hyaluronic acid gel • Silver nitrate pencil • CO_2 laser (2–5 mW)
Systemic options	• For severe cases use to supplement topical treatment strategies • Sucralfate • Colchicine • Pentoxifylline • Prednisolone and combinations[a]
Measures of effective treatment	• Relieves pain • Lessens functional impairment • Reduces frequency and severity of recurrences[d]

[a] Data from Descroix et al.[31]
[b] Data from Porter and Scully Cbe.[32]
[c] Data from Altenburg et al.[33]
[d] Data from Altenburg et al.[30]

Angioedema (Swelling)

(ACE inhibitors are the most prescribed class of hypertension and heart failure medications, accounting for approximately 35% of antihypertensive prescriptions in the United States.[34] Although rare (0.7%), severe adverse drug effects, such as angioedema, can occur.[35]

The accumulation of bradykinins results in ACE-inhibitor angioedema and is usually slower in onset than histamine-mediated angioedema. Swelling may involve different body organs, and in the orofacial area, the lips and tongue are the most common compromised locations. With the potential risk of limiting the airway, angioedema can be life threatening (**Fig. 2**). Most cases occur within the first 3 months of initiating the medication[36] (**Table 3**).

Dysesthesias (Altered Taste)

Alteration in taste
Medications have the potential to alter taste perception, although these mechanisms are not well understood. One belief is that drugs may alter the concentration of trace

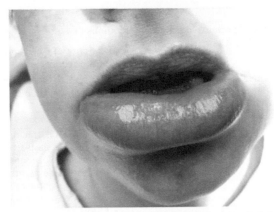

Fig. 2. Angioedema. (*Courtesy of* Dr. Mohammed Nadimul Islam, D.D.S., B.D.S, Florida.)

metals or alter receptors involved with taste and smell.[24] Research has identified in some cases that loss of taste in geriatric populations may result from physiologic changes in the cells initiating taste perception, declining olfactory function, poor nutrition, certain diseases, medications, and inadequate dentition.[38] Adverse drug reactions that affect taste include distortion of taste (dysgeusia), loss of ability to perceive certain taste sensations (hypogeusia), and loss of taste sensation (ageusia).[24]

Dysgeusia (altered sense of taste) is often seen in older patients because of chronic disease and polypharmacy, as well as physiologic, psychosocial, and emotional stress that can contribute to poor nutrition. Dysgeusia is further worsened by habits, such as tobacco and alcohol use, both of which cause an alteration in salivary flow, resulting in xerostomia.[39] Patients may seek relief by sucking hard candy as a way to mitigate the metallic taste and the lack of saliva, which lowers the pH in the saliva,

Table 3 Management strategies: angioedema	
Clinical presentation	• Abrupt onset of orofacial swelling may be life threatening if airway obstructed • Request emergency medical assistance immediately • Typically, if swelling is in front of maxillary teeth, drug treatment will be sufficient • If swelling is behind teeth, consider mechanical airway management[a]
Risk factors considerations	• Abrupt onset of swelling can be a *life-threatening emergency* because of potential for airway obstruction • Immediately request emergency medical assistance
Pharmaceutical recommendations	• Treat histamine-mediated angioedema with antihistamines (H1 and H2 antagonists)[b] • Combine oral corticosteroids along with epinephrine, as appropriate

[a] Data from Bernstein et al.[36]
[b] Data from Greaves and Lawlor.[37]

increasing caries risk. Alterations in taste significantly affect quality of life and can negatively affect diet choices and nutritional standing (**Table 4**).

Glossodynia (burning mouth syndrome)
Common systemic diseases and polypharmacy combinations used to manage conditions in aged populations have overlapping risk factors for burning mouth syndrome (BMS).[5] Worldwide, prevalence ranges from 1% to 4.8%, and it occurs in both men and women, with the latter being predisposed at a ratio of 6:1.[40]

BMS presents as burning sensations within the oral cavity (ie, tongue, lips, and oral mucosa) that are continuous and increase in intensity throughout the day.[5] The greatest frequency occurs on the anterior one-third of the tongue, followed by the gingiva and palate. Up to 50% of cases report concomitant xerostomia and dysgeusia, and the latter may be a result of a dysfunction of the sensory input to the tongue (ie, chorda tympani nerve).[40,41] This condition is likely of multifactorial origin, often idiopathic, and its etiopathogenesis remains largely enigmatic. In the scientific community, there is no consensus on the diagnosis or classification for BMS.[41] More often, it is a diagnosis of exclusion and may be associated with other oral manifestations, such as fungal infections and lichen planus, and may be exacerbated by nutritional deficiencies[5] (**Table 5**).

Oral candidiasis is the most observed oral fungal infection by dental providers (**Fig. 3**). In healthy adult populations, 30% to 60% have a species of *Candida* present in the oral cavity; most of these are not pathogenic but rather colonizing microorganisms.[42]

Pseudomembranous Candidiasis

Pseudomembranous candidiasis is the typical presentation of oral candidiasis, more commonly known as "thrush." One-third or more of all cases present as pseudomembranous candidiasis, with confluent white plaques on the tongue, buccal mucosa, hard palate, soft palate, and oral pharynx.[43,44] Classically, patients are asymptomatic. If symptoms develop, most are described as a burning oral sensation, altered taste, a sour taste, or propensity for bleeding. These lesions may be acute or chronic and are caused by the overgrowth of yeast in the oral mucosa with epithelial cell desquamation and accumulation of keratin, fibrin, necrotic tissue, and fungal hyphae.[45] A characteristic indicator for this candidiasis is the ability for the white plaques to be wiped off with gauze, exposing an erythematous surface (**Table 6**).

Fibrovascular Hyperplasia

Gingival hyperplasia develops mainly as an adverse effect from the treatment with certain antiepileptic, immunosuppressant, or antihypertensive medications. The 3 most studied classes of drugs include anticonvulsants (phenytoin),

Table 4	
Management strategies: dysesthesias: taste alterations	
Therapeutic recommendations	• Diet and nutritional counseling
Risk factors considerations	• Smoking • Alcohol consumption • High-sugar diet (compensate for alterations in taste perception) • Hard-candy consumption
Nutritional recommendations	• Mediterranean style diet • Xylitol lozenges to replace hard candy

Table 5 Management strategies: burning mouth syndrome	
Therapeutic options	• Patient education • Anxiety management • Short-term supportive psychotherapy • Cognitive behavioral therapy[a]
Risk factors considerations	• Polypharmacy • Maybe associated with fungal infection or lichen planus • Nutritional deficiencies • Systemic diseases
Pharmaceutical recommendations	• Central neuromodulators (tricyclic antidepressants, serotonin and norepinephrine reuptake inhibitors, selective serotonin reuptake inhibitors, clonazepam)[a]
Measures of effective treatment	• Because of variances in underlying conditions, there is no consensus on an effective treatment of all cases of BMS

[a] Data from Tu et al.[40]

immunosuppressants (cyclosporine), and various calcium channel blockers (nifedi-pine, verapamil, diltiazem).[49] Gingival hyperplasia has also been reported following the use of amlodipine,[49,50] verapamil,[51] and diltiazem.[52,53] Drug-induced gingival hyperplasia usually occurs within the first 3 months of starting the medication and begins as an enlargement of the interdental papilla.[54]

Gingival hyperplasia is characterized by an accumulation of extracellular matrix within the gingival connective tissue, particularly the collagenous components.[55] The excess gingival tissue has a negative impact on oral health, obstructing mastication, speech, and poor esthetics. Because of the gingival overgrowth, oral hygiene is compromised, predisposing the patient for periodontal disease.

Calcineurin inhibitors, such as cyclosporine, or less frequently, tacrolimus, also induce inflammatory fibrovascular hyperplasia in the oral cavity.[56] Conversely, these present as localized polypoid fibrous tumors and are often seen on the tongue and buccal mucosa rather than on the gingiva.[23]

Xerostomia (Dry Mouth)/Salivary Hypofunction

Dry mouth is one of the most common adverse effects of medication use in older adults.[11,57] Dry mouth includes salivary gland hypofunction (objectively measured

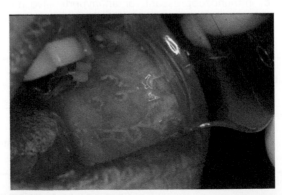

Fig. 3. Oral candidiasis. (*Courtesy of* Dr. Mohammed Nadimul Islam, D.D.S., B.D.S, Florida.)

Table 6 Management strategies: oral candidiasis	
Therapeutic considerations	• Underlying cause/risk factors must be removed • Mild cases may respond to topical antifungal treatment alone • Disease resistance/risk of disseminated candidiasis/immunocompromised will require systemic antifungal therapy
Risk factors considerations	• Immunocompromised (HIV/AIDS) • Immunosuppressed (tissue or organ transplant recipients, medications) • History of radiotherapy • Poor oral hygiene • Ill-fitting dental prosthesis • Nutritional deficiencies • Endocrine alterations (diabetes mellitus, renal failure, and hyperthyroidism) • Prolonged hospitalizations • Salivary gland hypofunction • Prolonged broad-spectrum use of antibiotics, topical steroids, and inhalers
Most common topical antifungal medications	• Gentian violet • Nystatin • Amphotericin B and imidazoles (miconazole, ketoconazole, and clotrimazole)
Most common systemic antifungal medications	• Oral fluconazole • Itraconazole • Posaconazole • Ketoconazole (NOTE: Food and Drug Administration advises against oral use due to the potential for hepatotoxicity in addition to drug interactions and adrenal insufficiency)

Data from Refs.[45–48]

decrease in salivation) and xerostomia (subjective feeling of dry mouth). It has been shown that the prevalence of hyposalivation increases with the number of medications used.[11] In a recent review, xerostomia was a commonly reported adverse oral effect associated with more than 80% of the one hundred most prescribed medications in the United States.[57] Although more than five hundred medications list dry mouth as an adverse effect, in controlled clinical trials, few have proven to affect salivary function.[58,59]

Decreased salivation is recurrently observed with anticholinergic medications, as well as with sympathomimetics, antidepressants, sedative hypnotics, opiates, antipsychotics, muscarinic receptor and α-receptor antagonists, antihypertensives (ie, diuretics, β-blockers, and ACE inhibitors), bronchodilators, antihistamines, and muscle relaxants.[55] Other medications include chemotherapy agents, appetite suppressants, decongestants, antimigraine drugs, opioids, benzodiazepines, hypnotics, histamine 2 (H2) receptor antagonists and proton pump inhibitors, systemic retinoid, HIV medications, and cytokine therapy.[57]

Xerostomia also occurs without changes in salivary flow rate, notably with psychological conditions, such as anxiety and depression, and following use of inhaled medications. More than 500 medications are associated with adverse effects on the salivary glands.[57]

Patients with chronic hyposalivation are highly susceptible to infections, such as candidiasis and bacterial sialadenitis. Because saliva acts as lubricant in the oral cavity, it plays a major role in the buffering capacities, when lacking can result in high caries risk (**Fig. 4**). The loss of lubrication also results in problems for denture patients, resulting in lack of retention and erythema owing to susceptibility of the mucosa to frictional trauma with profound discomfort and burning[60] (**Table 7**).

Because lack of saliva is a risk factor for a multitude of other conditions in the oral cavity, patient counseling is an ongoing task (**Table 8**).

Caries (decay) risk

Patients with chronic hyposalivation owing to medications are at risk for demineralization and dental cavitation (dental caries), often presenting as a severe form of rapidly developing decay that results in loss of dentition.[65] The lack of saliva and buffers creates an acidic environment suitable for dental demineralization and subsequently dental caries (**Fig. 5**). Another caries risk factor common in aged populations is root surface exposure owing to apical migration of the gingival margin. Cognitive, medical, and physical impairments are significant contributors to rapid deterioration of oral

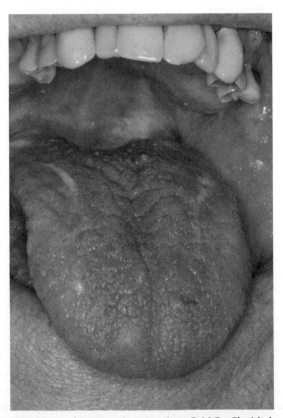

Fig. 4. Xerostomia. (*Courtesy of* Dr. Pamela R Sandow, D.M.D., Florida.)

Table 7 Management strategies: xerostomia	
Therapeutic considerations	• Increase other medical providers' awareness of signs, symptoms, and risk factors • Consult with prescribers to identify and alter (change or reduce dose) medications causing xerostomia • Patient education about protective role of saliva
Risk factors considerations	• Polypharmacy • Multimorbidities • Lack of saliva is a risk factor for several other conditions
Emerging research trends	• Botulinum toxin[a] • Systemic growth factors • Producing regenerative salivary gland tissue through transplantation or gene therapy • Tempol, a radioprotective agent[b]

[a] Data from Zaraa et al.[61]
[b] Data from Teymoortash et al.[62]

hygiene and associated increases in coronal and root caries. Although gingival recession and root caries may not be physiologic age alterations, clear evidence suggests prevalence of both increases with age.

Dysphagia (difficulty swallowing) Oropharyngeal dysphagia is widespread among older adults. Declines in salivary flow rates have been associated with reduced masticatory function. Subsequently, community-dwelling residents with impaired masticatory function have a high risk of malnutrition, frailty, and mortality.[66]

Dysphagia may lead to reduced food and fluid intake, with negative consequences of malnutrition, increased risk of aspiration, and aspiration pneumonia, which is cause

Table 8 Homecare strategies for xerostomia	
Homecare	**In Office**
Nutritional counseling	Caries risk assessment tools and sialometric tests
Oral moisturizers in sprays	Regular professionally applied chlorhexidine
Increase water intake	Silver diamine fluoride
Exposure to fluoridated rinses	Restoration with fluoride-releasing dental materials for active caries lesions
Avoid caffeine, alcohol, crunchy, spicy, acidic, or hard foods	Regular preventive-oriented recall appointments
Sialogogues (pharmacologic salivary production stimulants)	In-office topical fluoride applications
Saliva substitutes (artificial saliva) in mouthwashes or in gel	New: intraoral electrostimulation[a]
Xylitol lozenges to avoid hard candy	Hyperbaric oxygen[b]
Interproximal oral hygiene	Oral pilocarpine and cevimeline

[a] Data from Alajbeg et al.[63]
[b] Data from Teguh et al.[64]

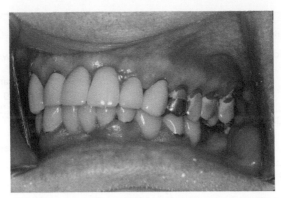

Fig. 5. Radiation caries. (*Courtesy of* Dr. Pamela R Sandow, D.M.D., Florida.)

for immediate and serious concern among frail older patients, especially those with limited or no access to medical care. One popular no-cost approach used in institutionalized patients is the Frazier free water protocol. Those with dysphagia who are prescribed modified diets (thick liquids or nothing by mouth) access thin (unthickened) water in between mealtimes. Specific guidelines are used to reduce risk of developing aspiration pneumonia. Limited evidence suggests that fluid intake may improve patients' perception of swallow-related quality of life.[67]

Lichenoid Reaction/Lichen Planus

Oral lichen planus (OLP) is a chronic inflammatory oral mucosal disease with a prevalence rate of 1% to 2%. OLP is frequently diagnosed in middle-aged and older female patients, with a female-to-male ratio of 1:5.[68] Medications for systemic diseases can cause oral lichenoid drug reaction.

The onset of OLP has been linked to ACE inhibitors, statins, Chinese herbal medicine, psoralen-UV-A therapy, and viral infection (varicella zoster virus).[61] Other suggested medications include active thiol groups found in the chemical structure of such medications as piroxicam, sulfasalazine, and glipizide, which play a role in inciting such reactions.[69]

Both reticular and atrophic/erosive OLP are related in oral lichenoid drug reaction. The time interval between administration of a certain medication to the onset of oral lichenoid drug reaction varies from weeks to a year or more. It usually presents as a single oral lesion, unlike the bilateral, symmetric, and multifocal presentations lesions[70] (**Fig. 6**). OLP presents as white striations or papules often associated with erythema or erosion and ulcers, most commonly in a bilaterally symmetric manner, often on the buccal mucosa, tongue, and gingiva[71] (**Fig. 7**).

If the drug causing the oral lichenoid drug reaction is identified, consult with the prescriber to discontinue the prescription and consider alternative options. Despite ceasing medication, it may take several months or longer for resolution of oral lesions. The histopathologic features of oral lichenoid medication reaction look like those of OLP. However, a more diffuse lymphocytic infiltrate mixed with plasma cells and eosinophils is observed. Moreover, the inflammatory infiltrate frequently extends to deeper connective tissue layers, and a perivascular inflammatory cell infiltration is often observed.[69]

Oral lichenoid lesions can be caused by dental materials and flavoring substances. The most reported dental restorative materials to cause oral lichenoid contact hypersensitivity reactions are amalgam, metals, composite resins, and glass ionomers and

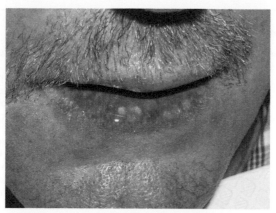

Fig. 6. OLP. (*Courtesy of* Dr. Mohammed Nadimul Islam, D.D.S., B.D.S, Florida.)

flavoring agents: cinnamon, eugenol, menthol, and peppermint. Dental material–induced oral lesions are most frequently found on the buccal mucosa and/or the lateral border of the tongue contacting the dental restoration.[70] Clinical studies have proven that the replacement of the dental restorations adjacent to these lesions is associated with healing, particularly when lesions are in close contact with restorations[72] (**Table 9**).

Osteonecrosis of Jaw

Osteonecrosis of the jaw is rare and initially was widely associated with bisphosphonate therapy and radiotherapy. New findings also link it with various antiresorptive therapies and antiangiogenic medications.[73] It can occur randomly but is often linked

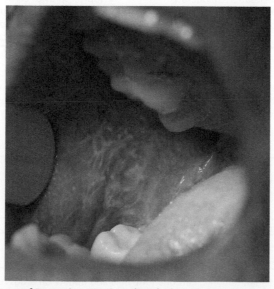

Fig. 7. OLP. (*Courtesy of* Dr. Mohammed Nadimul Islam, D.D.S., B.D.S, Florida.)

Table 9 Management strategies: lichenoid reaction/lichen planus	
Clinical presentation	• Nonerosive OLP (reticular, papular, or plaquelike lesion) • Nonerosive OLP lacks pain and burning sensation of oral mucosa upon eating hot, salty, acidic, or spicy food • Not necessary to treat nonerosive OLP lesions immediately • Erosive OLP (atrophic/erosive, ulcerative, or bullous lesion) includes oral symptoms, such as pain, burning sensation, and inflammation • Immediate and effective drug treatments should be offered for erosive OLP • Erosive OLP is an immunologically mediated disease
Therapeutic considerations	• Treatment depends on severity of symptoms • For medication induced, attempt to identify and consult with prescriber to alter • Results of discontinuing medication may not be apparent for months • Histopathologic features of oral lichenoid drug reaction look like those of OLP
Treatment recommendations: mild erosive OLP (small lesion, minimal symptoms)	• Topical application of corticosteroid (dexamethasone or triamcinolone) ointment • Apply as a thin film 2 or 3 times per day for 2 weeks
Treatment recommendations: moderate/severe erosive OLP (large lesion, increased symptoms)	• Topical spray of corticosteroid powders (ie, sealcoat cap for spray with beclomethasone dipropionate), apply to the lesion and mucosal areas

Data from Refs.[68,70,71]

Table 10 Medication-related osteonecrosis of jaw, relative risk, by medication type	
Medication	Relative Risk, %
Intravenous bisphosphonates (zoledronate and pamidronate)	0.7–6.7
Antiresorptive drug, denosumab	0.7–1.9
Antiangiogenic drugs bevacizumab	0.2

Data from Eguia A, Bagán-Debón L, Cardona F. Review and update on drugs related to the development of osteonecrosis of the jaw. Med Oral Patol Oral Cir Bucal. 2020;25(1):e71-e83.

Table 11 Management strategies: medication-related osteonecrosis of jaw	
Clinical presentation	• Stages (0–3) progressive from no bony exposure (1/3 of all cases), asymptomatic bony exposure, to pain, inflammation, loose teeth, infection, contained within and outside of the dentoalveolar area • Occurs in maxilla or mandible, more prevalent in latter
Therapeutic considerations	• No cure, prevention is critical • Requires constant awareness of new medications
Risk factors considerations	• Intravenous bisphosphonates (zoledronate and pamidronate) • Antiresorptive drug, denosumab • Antiangiogenic drugs bevacizumab • Risedronate, ibandronate, and alendronate • TKI inhibitor (sunitinib) • Polypharmacy with corticoids • Morbidities such as diabetes

Data from Refs.[73–75]

with oral surgery and identified pharmacologic treatments.[74] Broader association with different medications has altered nomenclature from bisphosphonate-related osteonecrosis of jaw to medication-related osteonecrosis of jaw (MROJN). Its defined as one or more exposed bone lesions in the oral cavity for 8 weeks or more, with current or past history of treatment with antiresorptive and/or antiangiogenic agents without the presence of radiotherapy, which is now classified separately from MROJN.[73,75] Importantly, this definition does not properly describe the nonexposed bone variant, which accounts for one-third of all MROJN cases.[73] MROJN can occur in either than maxilla or the mandible but is more prevalent in the latter.[74] Exact pathogenesis is still inconclusive; common theories include reduced bone remodeling, presence of

Box 3 Step-by-step systematic dental polypharmacy assessment and medication reconciliation
Step One: Obtain patient medical and dental history via questionnaire
Step Two: Conduct patient interview
Step Three: Review patient's medical history, medications, over-the- counter medications, dietary/herbal supplements and verify (dose, frequency, route, and compliance) for accuracy and completeness
Step Four: Assess any patient on multiple medications for risk factors of polypharmacy (see **Table 1**. Most prevalent risk factors for polypharmacy in older patients)
Step Five: Conduct medication reconciliation for any polypharmacy patient cases (see **Table 12**. Example of medical reconciliation and medication assessment)
Step Six: Use a clinical pharmacologic information database to assess existing medications for impact on dental care, medication-induced oral implications, and potential adverse effects of any newly proposed prescriptions
Data from Reconcile Medications in Outpatient Settings. Institute for Healthcare Improvement. 2015. Available at: http://www.ihi.org/resources/Pages/Changes/ReconcileMedicationsinOut patientSettings.aspx. Accessed July 27,2020.

Table 12
Example of medical reconciliation and medication assessment

Diagnoses	Onset	Medication/Over the Counter/Herbal	Dosage	Laboratory Values	Notes (Safety, Redundant, Oral Contraindications)
1. Diabetes type II	1997	Metformin	500 mg tid	HBa1c 7% 7/10/2000	Medline Plus reports possibility of metallic taste[a]
2. Perpheral artery disease	2018	Clopidogrel	75 mg qd	Not available; information is not available or missing (ie, medications, regimens, laboratory values), a best practice is to consult with the prescriber to obtain	Excessive bleeding: oral surgery, per MD, cease medication 5 d prior
3. Hypertension	2019	Lisinopril	20 mg qd	Blood pressure 120/80	Xerostomia
4. Self-prescribed, for "concentration improvement"	2020	Ginkgo biloba	60 mg qd	None Request additional information for medications that lack a correlated systemic problem or condition	Consulted National Center for Collaborative Healthcare Innovation clearinghouse: increased risk of bleeding contraindicated with blood thinners; clopidogrel advised discontinuation[b]

Patient XXX. Date of medical history: 10/01/2000 Updated: 2018, 2019, 2020.
[a] Data from US National Library of Medicine.[76]
[b] Data from National Center for Complementary and Integrative Medicine.[77]

infection, angiogenesis, and dysfunctional innate and acquired immunity[73,75] **(Tables 10 and 11)**.

ASSESSMENT

The following section outlines a systematic, step-by-step assessment process and provides a template for medication reconciliation that can easily be integrated into dental clinical workflow (**Box 3**).

Medication reconciliation should be systematically applied to all patients and updated at each dental appointment. If any information is not available or missing (medications, regimens, laboratory values), best practice is to consult with the prescriber to obtain the missing information. Also, additional information should be requested for medications that lack a correlated systemic problem or condition (**Table 12**).

SUMMARY

Oral health care providers should be familiar with oral lesions related to a high prevalence of polypharmacy and multimorbidities in older patient populations. Manifestations of adverse drug events in the oral cavity are common. Clinical diagnosis and developing management strategies are critical to deliver effective treatment. With the discovery of new diseases and management strategies for chronic conditions, more adverse medication reactions will be encountered. It is also important to continuously raise awareness within the medical community regarding adverse medication-induced manifestations, as these oral lesions have an impact on our patient's quality of life.

CLINICS CARE POINTS

- It is critical to stay apprised of evidence-based, clinical pharmacologic knowledge to diagnose and treat oral implications of medications.
- Medication reconciliation is an effective tool to integrate into dental clinical practice to assure accurate medical information.
- Oral health providers must be cognizant of the risk factors of polypharmacy in older populations and regularly assess patients.
- Communicate treatment needs to other prescribers to reduce medication errors and inappropriate polypharmacy.

DISCLOSURE

The authors have nothing to disclose.

REFERENCES

1. He W, Goodkind D, Kowal PR. An aging world: 2015. Atlanta: Centers for Disease Control and Prevention; 2016. Available at: https://www.census.gov/content/dam/Census/library/publications/2016/demo/p95-16-1.pdf. Accessed July 17, 2020.
2. Centers for Disease Control and Prevention. 65 and older population grows rapidly as baby boomers age. Available at: https://www.census.gov/newsroom/press-releases/2020/65-older-population-grows.html. Accessed October 12, 2020.

3. Vespa J. The graying of America: more older adults than kids by 2035. United States Census Bureau. Available at: https://www.census.gov/library/stories/2018/03/graying-america.html. Accessed October 12, 2020.
4. World Health Organization. Medication safety in polypharmacy: technical report. 2019. Available at: https://apps.who.int/iris/bitstream/handle/10665/325454/WHO-UHC-SDS-2019.11-eng.pdf?ua=1. Accessed July 19,2020.
5. Halpern LR. The geriatric syndrome and oral health: navigating oral disease treatment strategies in the elderly. Dent Clin North Am Jan 2020;64(1):209–28.
6. Masnoon N, Shakib S, Kalisch-Ellett L, et al. What is polypharmacy? A systematic review of definitions. BMC Geriatr 2017;17(1):230.
7. Cadogan CA, Ryan C, Francis JJ, et al. Improving appropriate polypharmacy for older people in primary care: selecting components of an evidence-based intervention to target prescribing and dispensing. Implement Sci 2015;10(1):161.
8. Michocki RJ. Polypharmacy and principles of drug therapy. In: Adelman AM, Daly MP, editors. 20 common problems in geriatrics. New York: McGraw-Hill; 2001. p. 69–81.
9. Quinn KJ, Shah NH. A dataset quantifying polypharmacy in the United States. Sci Data 2017;4:170167.
10. Centers for Disease Control and Prevention, Health, United States, 2018, table 38. Available at: https://www.cdc.gov/nchs/data/hus/2018/038.pdf. Accessed July 9, 2020.
11. Johnell K, Fastbom J. Comparison of prescription drug use between community-dwelling and institutionalized elderly in Sweden. Drugs Aging 2012;29(9):751–8.
12. German PS, Burton LC. Medication and the elderly. Issues of prescription and use. J Aging Health 1989;1:4–34.
13. Atchison KA, Rozier RG, Weintraub JA. Integration of oral health and primary care: communication, coordination and referral. Washington, DC: NAM Perspectives; 2018.
14. Nam Y, Kim NH, Kho HS. Geriatric oral and maxillofacial dysfunctions in the context of geriatric syndrome. Oral Dis 2018;24(3):317–24.
15. Komiya H, Umegaki H, Asai A, et al. Factors associated with polypharmacy in elderly home-care patients. Geriatr Gerontol Int 2018;8(1):33–41.
16. Duke JD, Li X, Grannis SJ. Data visualization speeds review of potential adverse drug events in patients on multiple medications. J Biomed Inform 2010;43(2):326–31.
17. Fitzgerald J, Epstein JB, Mark Donaldson B, et al. Outpatient medication use and implications for dental care: guidance for contemporary dental practice. J Can Dent Assoc 2015;81:f10.
18. U.S. Department of Health and Human Services. Oral health in America: a report of the surgeon general. Rockville (MD): U.S. Department of Health and Human Services, National Institute of Dental and Craniofacial Research, National Institutes of Health; 2000. Available at: https://www.nidcr.nih.gov/research/data-statistics/surgeon-general.
19. Chapple I. The impact of oral disease upon systemic health-symposium overview. J dentistry 2009;37(8):S568.
20. Shinkai RS, Hatch JP, Schmidt CB, et al. Exposure to the oral side effects of medication in a community-based sample. Spec Care Dentist 2006;26(3):116–20.
21. Greiver M, Dahrouge S, O'Brien P, et al. Improving care for elderly patients living with polypharmacy: protocol for a pragmatic cluster randomized trial in community-based primary care practices in Canada. Implement Sci 2019;14(1):55.

22. Halli-Tierney AD, Scarbrough C, Carroll D. Polypharmacy: evaluating risks and deprescribing. Am Fam Physician 2019;100(1):32–8.
23. Yuan A, Woo SB. Adverse drug events in the oral cavity. Oral Surg Oral Med Oral Pathol Oral Radiol Jan 2015;119(1):35–47.
24. Spolarich AE. Risk management strategies for reducing oral adverse drug events. J Evid Based Dental Pract 2014;14:87–94.e1.
25. Shah K, Guarderas J, Krishnaswamy G. Aphthous stomatitis. Ann Allergy Asthma Immunol 2016;117(4):341–3.
26. Boulinguez S, Reix S, Bedane C, et al. Role of drug exposure in aphthous ulcers: a case-control study. Br J Dermatol 2000;143:1261–5.
27. Muñoz-Corcuera M, Esparza-Gómez G, González-Moles M, et al. Oral ulcers: clinical aspects. A tool for dermatologists. Part II. Chronic ulcers. Clin Exp Dermatol Clin Dermatol 2009;34(4):456–61.
28. Pisano U, Deosaran J, Leslie SJ, et al. Nicorandil, gastrointestinal adverse drug reactions and ulcerations: a systematic review. Adv Ther 2016;33(3):320–44.
29. Abdollahi M, Radfar M. A review of drug-induced oral reactions. J Contemp Dent Pract 2003;4(1):10–31.
30. Altenburg A, El-Haj N, Micheli C, et al. The treatment of chronic recurrent oral aphthous ulcers. Dtsch Arztebl Int 2014;111(40):665–73.
31. Descroix V, Coudert AE, Vigé A, et al. Efficacy of topical 1% lidocaine in the symptomatic treatment of pain associated with oral mucosal trauma or minor oral aphthous ulcer: a randomized, double-blind, placebo-controlled, parallel-group, single-dose study. J Orofac Pain 2011;25:327–32.
32. Porter SR, Scully Cbe C. Aphthous ulcers (recurrent). BMJ Clin Evid 2007;2007: 1303.
33. Altenburg A, Abdel-Naser MB, Abdallah M, et al. Practical aspects of management of recurrent aphthous stomatitis. J Eur Acad Dermatol Venereol 2007;21: 1019–26.
34. Ma J, Lee K-V, Stafford RS. Changes in antihypertensive prescribing during US outpatient visits for uncomplicated hypertension between 1993 and 2004. Hypertension 2006;48(5):846–52.
35. Banerji A, Blumenthal KG, Lai KH, et al. Epidemiology of ACE inhibitor angioedema utilizing a large electronic health record. J Allergy Clin Immunol 2017; 5(3):744–9.
36. Bernstein JA, Cremonesi P, Hoffmann TK, et al. Angioedema in the emergency department: a practical guide to differential diagnosis and management. Int J Emerg Med 2017;10(1):15.
37. Greaves M, Lawlor F. Angioedema: manifestations and management. J Am Acad Dermatol 1991;25(1):155–65.
38. Sergi G, Bano G, Pizzato S, et al. Taste loss in the elderly: possible implications for dietary habits. Crit Rev Food Sci Nutr 2017;57(17):3684–9.
39. Pisano M, Hilas O. Zinc and taste disturbances in older adults: a review of the literature. Consult Pharm 2016;31(5):267–70.
40. Tu TT, Takenoshita M, Matsuoka H, et al. Current management strategies for the pain of elderly patients with burning mouth syndrome: a critical review. BioPsychoSocial Med 2019;13(1):1.
41. Scala A, Checchi L, Montevecchi M, et al. Update on burning mouth syndrome: overview and patient management. Crit Rev Oral Biol Med 2003;14(4):275–91.
42. Hellstein JW, Marek CL. Candidiasis: red and white manifestations in the oral cavity. Head Neck Pathol 2019;13(1):25–32.
43. Akpan A, Morgan R. Oral candidiasis. Postgrad Med J 2002;78(922):455–9.

44. Muzyka BC. Oral fungal infections. Dental Clin 2005;49(1):49–65.
45. Sharon V, Fazel N. Oral candidiasis and angular cheilitis. Dermatol Ther 2010; 23(3):230–42.
46. Patton LL. Oral lesions associated with human immunodeficiency virus disease. Dental Clin 2013;57(4):673–98.
47. Coronado-Castellote L, Jiménez-Soriano Y. Clinical and microbiological diagnosis of oral candidiasis. J Clin Exp Dent 2013;5(5):e279–86.
48. Millsop JW, Fazel N. Oral candidiasis. Clin Dermatol 2016;34(4):487–94.
49. Goriuc A, Foia LG, Minea B, et al. Drug-induced gingival hyperplasia-experimental model. Rom J Morphol Embryol 2017;58(4):1371–6.
50. Seymour R, Ellis J, Thomason J, et al. Amlodipine-induced gingival overgrowth. J Clin Periodontol 1994;21(4):281–3.
51. Bhatia V, Mittal A, Parida AK, et al. Amlodipine induced gingival hyperplasia: a rare entity. Int J Cardiol 2007;122(3):e23–4.
52. Seymour R, Smith D. The effect of a plaque control programme on the incidence and severity of cyclosporin-induced gingival changes. J Clin Periodontol 1991; 18(2):107–10.
53. Bowman JM, Levy BA, Grubb RV. Gingival overgrowth induced by diltiazem: a case report. Oral Surg Oral Med Oral Pathol 1988;65(2):183–5.
54. Fattore L, Stablein M, Bredfeldt G, et al. Gingival hyperplasia: a side effect of nifedipine and diltiazem. Spec Care Dentist 1991;11(3):107–9.
55. Nishikawa S, Nagata T, Morisaki I, et al. Pathogenesis of drug-induced gingival overgrowth. A review of studies in the rat model. J Periodontol 1996;67(5): 463–71.
56. Yamasaki A, Rose G, Pinero G, et al. Ultrastructure of fibroblasts in cyclosporin A-induced gingival hyperplasia. J Oral Pathol Med 1987;16(3):129–34.
57. Scully C. Drug effects on salivary glands: dry mouth. Oral Dis 2003;9:165–76.
58. Femiano F, Rullo R, di Spirito F, et al. A comparison of salivary substitutes versus a natural sialogogue (citric acid) in patients complaining of dry mouth as an adverse drug reaction: a clinical, randomized controlled study. Oral Surg Oral Med Oral Pathol Oral Radiol Endodontology. 2011;112(1):e15–20.
59. Zavras AI, Rosenberg GE, Danielson JD, et al. Adverse drug and device reactions in the oral cavity: surveillance and reporting. J Am Dent Assoc Sep 2013; 144(9):1014–21.
60. Millsop JW, Wang EA, Fazel N. Etiology, evaluation, and management of xerostomia. Clin Dermatol 2017;35(5):468–76.
61. Zaraa I, Mahfoudh A, Sellami MK, et al. Lichen planus pemphigoides: four new cases and a review of the literature. Int J Dermatol 2013;52(4):406–12.
62. Teymoortash Ax, Muller F, Juricko J, et al. Botulinum toxin prevents radiotherapy-induced salivary gland damage. Oral Oncol 2009;45:737–9.
63. Alajbeg I, Falcão DP, Tran SD, et al. Intraoral electrostimulator for xerostomia relief: a long-term, multicenter, open-label, uncontrolled, clinical trial. Oral Surg Oral Med Oral Pathol Oral Radiol 2012;113(6):773–81.
64. Teguh DN, Levendag PC, Noever I, et al. Early hyperbaric oxygen therapy for reducing radiotherapy side effects: early results of a randomized trial in oropharyngeal and nasopharyngeal cancer. Int J Radiat Oncol Biol Phys 2009;75(3): 711–6.
65. Deng J, Jackson L, Epstein JB, et al. Dental demineralization and caries in patients with head and neck cancer. Oral Oncol 2015;51(9):824–31.
66. Barbe AG. Medication-induced xerostomia and hyposalivation in the elderly: culprits, complications, and management. Drugs Aging 2018;35(10):877–85.

67. Gillman A, Winkler R, Taylor NF. Implementing the free water protocol does not result in aspiration pneumonia in carefully selected patients with dysphagia: a systematic review. Dysphagia 2017;32(3):345–61.
68. Cheng Y-SL, Gould A, Kurago Z, et al. Diagnosis of oral lichen planus: a position paper of the American Academy of Oral and Maxillofacial Pathology. Oral Surg Oral Med Oral Pathol Oral Radiol 2016;122(3):332–54.
69. Breathnach S. Mechanisms of drug eruptions: part I. Australas J Dermatol 1995; 36(3):121–7.
70. Chiang C-P, Chang JY-F, Wang Y-P, et al. Oral lichen planus–differential diagnoses, serum autoantibodies, hematinic deficiencies, and management. J Formos Med Assoc 2018;117(9):756–65.
71. Piboonniyom S-o, Treister N, Pitiphat W, et al. Scoring system for monitoring oral lichenoid lesions: a preliminary study. Oral Surg Oral Med Oral Pathol Oral Radiol Endodontology 2005;99(6):696–703.
72. Issa Y, Duxbury A, Macfarlane T, et al. Oral lichenoid lesions related to dental restorative materials. Br Dent J 2005;198(6):361–6.
73. Omolehinwa TT, Akintoye SO. Chemical and radiation-associated jaw lesions. Dent Clin North Am 2016;60(1):265–77.
74. Eguia A, Bagán-Debón L, Cardona F. Review and update on drugs related to the development of osteonecrosis of the jaw. Med Oral Patol Oral Cir Bucal 2020; 25(1):e71–83.
75. Rugani P, Walter C, Kirnbauer B, et al. Prevalence of medication-related osteonecrosis of the jaw in patients with breast cancer, prostate cancer, and multiple myeloma. Dent J (Basel) 2016;4(4):32.
76. Metformin. Medline Plus. U.S. National Library of Medicine. 2020. Available at: https://medlineplus.gov/druginfo/meds/a696005.html. Accessed July 25, 2020.
77. Ginko. National Center for Complementary and Integrative Medicine. U.S. Department of Health and Human Services. 2016. Available at: https://www.nccih.nih.gov/health/ginkgo. Accessed July 25, 2020.

Cognitive Impairment in Older Adults and Oral Health Considerations

Treatment and Management

Paul S. Farsai, DMD, MPH[a,b]

KEYWORDS

- Cognitive impairment • Oral health • Dental treatment • Dental management

KEY POINTS

- Variations in cognitive impairment in patients cause behavioral changes in patients which may then affect the ability to provide and maintain dental care.
- The proper diagnosis for cognitive impairment and knowledge of available medical treatment modalities allow for a better understanding of the systemic interactions with the dental care.
- Practitioners should be well aware of the process of informed consent since cognitively impaired patients are unable to consent to or approve oral care.
- Dental maintenance and management after treatment should continue on within an interdisciplinary approach.

INTRODUCTION

Cognitive impairment (CI) in older adults is a broad term for a variety of functions and activities that effect memory recall, learning, concentration, or decision-making skills occurring in the elderly.[1]

There are several degrees and levels of CI, ranging from mild CI (MCI) to dementia. Although at one point all were grouped into a single condition as part of the natural aging process, research shows each as unique, with different causes, symptoms, and treatment.[2]

It is now estimated that the over–65-year-old age group constitutes approximately 15% of the US population.[3,4] Despite the increase in multiple chronic conditions (MCCs) with age, most people with MCCs now are individuals younger than 65 years old.[4] To some investigators, the high rate of CI among younger adults with MCCs may

This article originally appeared in Dental Clinics, Volume 65 Issue 2, April 2021.
P.S. Farsai has no conflicts of interest to disclose.
[a] Department of General Dentistry, Boston University, Henry M. Goldman School of Dental Medicine, 72 East Concord Street, Robinson Room 334, Boston, MA 02118-2526, USA; [b] Private dental practice, Swampscott, MA, USA
E-mail address: pfarsai@bu.edu

be a somewhat unexpected finding. This could be a result, however, of lower rates of other chronic conditions or factors, such as lack of sleep, side effects of medication, and use of illicit drugs, and may not be associated with future risk of dementia. Whatever the cause, being cognitively impaired may affect someone's ability to self-manage other chronic conditions. In 2017, the US Centers for Disease Control and Prevention reported that those individuals younger than age 65 were more likely to report asthma, CI, depression, smoking, obesity, poorer access to health care, disability, and worse quality of life than those adults age 65 or older with MCCs.[4] Based on these reports, it was estimated that the future risk of CI is approximately 28.6% for the greater than 65-year-old category compared with 57.2% in the less than 65-year-old category. These estimates for the less than 65-year-old cohort paint a picture that many more CI issues may have to be addressed in the future than currently are addressed today.

Age remains the greatest risk factor for CI, and, as the baby boomer generation passes age 65, the number of people living with CI is expected to jump dramatically.[5] An estimated 5.1 million Americans age 65 years or older currently may have Alzheimer disease, the most well-known form of CI; this number may rise to 13.2 million by 2050.[6] CI is costly. People with CI report more than 3 times as many hospital stays as individuals who are hospitalized for some other condition. Alzheimer disease and related dementias alone are estimated to be the third most expensive disease to treat in the United States.

As the impairment develops, a person may notice changes in their cognitive function but still have success accomplishing everyday activities and living independently. More severe types of impairment can affect a person's ability to control bodily movements and manual dexterity and understand the meaning or importance of something as well as affecting speech and writing abilities. Therefore, when treating older adults, it is important to understand that oral health issues relevant to the healthy aging population are different than those who are aging with impairments or disabilities because providers have to bear in mind that oral health needs to be managed and maintained in concert with a patient's impairments.[7]

COGNITION AND DAILY LIVING

Professionals who work in aging often want to know whether an older person needs any help with activities of daily living (ADLs) and instrumental ADLs (IADLs). As discussed in Joseph M. Calabrese and Kadambari Rawal' article,"*Demographics and Oral Health Care Utilization for Older Adults*" in this issue, they represent key life tasks that people need to manage in order to live at home and be fully independent.

Difficulties with ADLs and IADLs often correspond to how much help, supervision, and hands-on care an older person needs to obtain in order to be comfortable, functional, and safe. This assessment can determine the cost of care at a facility, whether someone is considered safe to live at home, or even whether a person is eligible for long-term care services. For each ADL, people can vary from needing just a little help (such as a reminder or a person to stand-by assist) to full dependency, which requires others to do a task for them.[8,9]

WHY ACTIVITIES OF DAILY LIVING AND INDEPENDENT ACTIVITIES OF DAILY LIVING MATTER

Generally, older adults need to be able to manage ADLs and IADLs in order to live independently without the assistance of another person. Periodic assessment of ADLs and IADLs as part of the ongoing assessment of an older person's function typically reveals problems with physical health, cognitive health, or both. Identifying functional difficulties can help medical and dental practitioners diagnose and manage important overall health and oral problems.

Identification of functional difficulties also is crucial because medical providers want to make sure older adults are getting the help and support they need to compensate for or overcome the functional difficulties. In doing so, any family caregivers who might be struggling to assist a relative who needs help can become aware of addressing these issues with the health care team.

More importantly, if a person is not fully independent with ADLs and IADLs, then the oral health provider should ask the nursing home staff, visiting nurse, caretaker, or family member to include some information about the amount of assistance they require. These individuals serve as resources and can help the oral health team to facilitate the formulation of a dental treatment plan as well as a maintenance program that becomes more realistic and achievable.

GERIATRIC EVALUATION OVERVIEW

Geriatric assessments provide a valuable basis for evaluating treatment decisions and the prediction of treatment tolerance in the elderly. Geriatric assessments in the dental setting may be more comprehensive than assessments done on other patients and usually cover the domains of general medical health as well as cognitive, social, and physical functions. They also should include evaluation of caregiver and environmental concerns, with an emphasis on the optimization of dependent or independent function.[9] A typical geriatric assessment in a dental setting should include the following components:

- Communication
- Physical
- Mobility
- Mental
- Nutritional
- Dental
- Social
- Medical

To aid practitioners, there are multiple performance-based screening tools designed for measuring cognitive issues in older adults, such as[10]

- Mini-Mental State Examination (MMSE)—the most common tool used
- Lawton IADL scale—analyzes functional ability; has a scale range of 0 to 9
- Katz ADL scale—has a scale range of 0 to 6
- Stanford Health Assessment Questionnaire 8-item Disability Index (HAQ 8-item DI)—the complete version of HAQ has 5 subscales and 1 of the subscales is the disability scale, which has been used frequently as an independent questionnaire.

All components of the geriatric assessment should be reviewed briefly at every dental visit, because they change more frequently in the cognitively impaired or frail elderly and can identify barriers to maintaining good oral health.

MILD COGNITIVE IMPAIRMENT

Cognitive decline is a common and often feared aspect of aging. Mild Cognitive Impairment (MCI) is defined as the "symptomatic pre-dementia stage" on the continuum from normal cognition to dementia, characterized by objective impairment in cognition that is not severe enough to require help with usual ADLs.[8,11] Unlike other types of CI that affect speech and bodily control, with MCI, only 1 function is declining—memory. A roadblock to earlier diagnosis and potential treatment is the lack of consistency with screening for MCI. Universal screening would be ideal but is limited (**Box 1**).

At present time, there are no pharmacologic treatments proved to slow or cure progression of MCI to dementia; nonetheless, there is evidence that lifestyle modifications, including diet, exercise, and cognitive stimulation, may be effective in postponing or managing early MCI symptoms. A person with MCI is at increased risk for developing more severe types of impairment like dementia or Alzheimer dementia.

Although patients with MCI are at greater risk of developing dementia compared with the general population, there currently is substantial variation in risk estimates (from <5% to 20% annual conversion rates), depending on the population studied. Risk typically increases with age, and men appear to be at higher risk than women.[10]

Critical features that may elucidate a cause are onset, trajectory, time course, and nature of the cognitive symptoms (**Box 2**).[2] Very rapid cognitive decline (eg, weeks to months) is not typical of MCI due to Alzheimer disease and should raise concerns for other causes, such as neoplasm, metabolic disorders, or prion disease. Patients and informants (such as family members) may report conflicting views regarding the presence and severity of cognitive symptoms, either from lack of insight or because cognitive decline can be emotionally charged and symptom report may be minimized to avoid difficult or disrespectful discussions.

DEMENTIA

Dementia is more severe than MCI, but initial symptoms appear in the same gradual and progressive manner. Approximately 5 million Americans are living with an age-related form of dementia, and it has been reported that approximately one-quarter are undiagnosed for quite some time. There are several types of dementia[12–16]:

- Vascular dementia is caused by an impaired blood supply to the brain and may be brought on by stroke.
- Dementia with Lewy bodies is linked to Alzheimer disease and Parkinson disease. It typically results from the death of nerve cells and loss of tissue in the brain.

Box 1
Screening for cognitive impairment: points to remember

- The person, family member, or others express concerns about changes in the patient's memory or thinking.
- Provider observe problems/changes in the patient's memory or thinking.
- The patient is age 80 or older, because the risk of dementia increases rapidly after this age.
- Other risk factors that could indicate the need for dementia screening include low education, history of type 2 diabetes mellitus, stroke, depression, and trouble managing money or medications.
- Various dementia screening methods are available and can be used.
- Patients who specifically express a concern likely want to know what the underlying problem is.

Barnes DE, Beiser AS, Lee A, et al. Development and validation of a brief dementia screening indicator for primary care. *Alzheimers Dement.* 2014;10(6):656-665.e1.

Box 2
Criteria for the diagnosis of mild cognitive impairment

1. Concern regarding a change in cognition from the patient, knowledgeable informant, or from a skilled clinician observing the patient

2. Objective evidence of impairment (from cognitive testing) in 1 or more cognitive domains, including memory, executive function, attention, language, or visuospatial skills

3. Preservation of independence in functional abilities (although individuals may be less efficient and make more errors at performing ADLs/IADLs than in the past)

4. No evidence of a significant impairment in social or occupational functioning (ie not demented)

Data from Albert MS, DeKosky ST, Dickson D, Dubois B, Feldman HH, Fox NC, Gamst A, Holtzman DM, Jagust WJ, Petersen RC, Snyder PJ, Carrillo MC, Thies B, Phelps CH. The diagnosis of mild cognitive impairment due to Alzheimer's disease: recommendations from the National Institute on Aging-Alzheimer's Association workgroups on diagnostic guidelines for Alzheimer's disease. Alzheimers Dement. 2011 May; 7(3):270-9.

- Frontotemporal dementia is a group of disorders triggered by gradual nerve cell loss in the brain's frontal and temporal lobes.

These are a small sample of many forms of dementia seen in the elderly.

ALZHEIMER DISEASE

Alzheimer disease is the most serious, and common, form of dementia. It is a progressive disease, with symptoms developing gradually before they intensify over time. In its late stages, the disease can make it difficult for a person to handle daily tasks, think clearly, control bodily movements, and live independently.[14,17] Alzheimer disease accounts for 60% to 80% of dementia cases and is the sixth leading cause of death in the United States. At the initial stage of the disease, forgetfulness and mild confusion are seen (**Box 3**).[2] Over time, recent memories also start erasing. Advanced stage symptoms vary from person to person, because there is no cure for Alzheimer disease.

Alzheimer disease has a complex etiology and is associated with genetic, lifestyle, and environmental factors that affect the brain cells over time[18] (**Box 4**). The loss of memory, especially for learning and retaining new information, reflects impaired function in the hippocampus and other medial temporal lobe structures, which are sites of early pathologic change.

Symptoms

As the disease progresses, the symptoms often manifest in more persistent language disturbance and difficulties completing more complex tasks of daily living. Patients progress from loss of higher-level IADLs, such as the ability to perform financial transactions and drive a car or use public transportation, to abnormalities in the more basic ADLs (personal hygiene or toileting). Behavioral problems frequently develop and include depression, apathy, anxiety, agitation, psychosis (delusions and hallucinations), wandering, and aggression (**Box 5**).

Treatment

Medications and nutrition are important as both causative and protective factors in Alzheimer disease. There appears to be a correlation between cognitive skills and the use of estrogen and anti-inflammatory drugs as well as serum concentrations of folate, vitamin B_{12}, vitamin B_6, and homocysteine.[19] Treatment of Alzheimer disease

---

Box 3
Clinical characteristics suggestive that mild cognitive impairment is due to Alzheimer disease

1. Memory impairment present

2. Progressive decline in cognition over months to years (very rapid decline may suggest prion disease, neoplasm, or metabolic disorders)

3. Lack of parkinsonism and visual hallucinations (suggestive of dementia with Lewy bodies)

4. Lack of vascular risk factors and extensive cerebrovascular disease on brain imaging (suggestive of vascular CI)

5. Lack of prominent behavioral or language disorders (suggestive of frontotemporal lobar degeneration)

Data from Albert MS, DeKosky ST, Dickson D, Dubois B, Feldman HH, Fox NC, Gamst A, Holtzman DM, Jagust WJ, Petersen RC, Snyder PJ, Carrillo MC, Thies B, Phelps CH. The diagnosis of mild cognitive impairment due to Alzheimer's disease: recommendations from the National Institute on Aging-Alzheimer's Association workgroups on diagnostic guidelines for Alzheimer's disease. Alzheimers Dement. 2011 May; 7(3):270-9.

---

is based on an accurate diagnosis, which often requires laboratory tests and imaging data.

Inhibition of acetylcholinesterase (ACE) currently is the most successful treatment of Alzheimer disease.[20,21] Unfortunately, however, ACE inhibitors (like other pharmacologic strategies) just slow down or delay the progression of the disease but ultimately do not stop or cure it. Other medications can reduce some symptoms temporarily or slow down the progression of the condition in some people (**Box 6**).

Among nonpharmacologic interventions for mild/moderate dementia, the recommendation is caregiver education, supportive therapy, and respite care for caregivers. For patients, it is referral to day treatment and exercise programs. For moderate/severe

---

Box 4
Alzheimer disease and causes

Background

- Very common (more than 3 million cases per year in the United States)

- Often requires laboratory test or imaging

- Treatments can help manage condition, no known cure

- Can last several years or be lifelong

Factors known to increase the risk of developing the condition
- Age
- Family history and genetics
- Down syndrome
- Head injuries
- Past head trauma
- MCI

Alzheimer disease causes shrinkage (atrophy) of the posterior part of the brain
- Amyloid plaques (abnormal deposits of protein) that damage and destroy brain cells
- Neurofibrillary tangles—brain cells require the normal structure and functioning of a protein called tau. In Alzheimer disease, threads of tau protein twist into abnormal tangles inside brain cells, leading to the death of brain cells.

Data from Hugo J, Ganguli M. Dementia and cognitive impairment: epidemiology, diagnosis, and treatment. Clin Geriatr Med. 2014;30(3):421-442.

Box 5
Alzheimer disease symptoms

Early-stage symptoms
• Memory loss
• Misplacing items
• Forgetting the names of places and objects
• Repeating themselves regularly, such as asking the same question several times
• Becoming less flexible and more hesitant to try new things

Middle-stage symptoms include
• Increasing confusion and disorientation
• Obsessive, repetitive, or impulsive behavior
• Delusions (believing things that are untrue)
• Problems with speech or language (aphasia)
• Disturbed sleep
• Changes in mood, such as frequent mood swings, depression, and feeling increasingly anxious, frustrated, or agitated
• Difficulty in performing spatial tasks, such as judging distances
• Agnosia

Later-stage symptoms include
• Difficulty in changing position or moving around without assistance
• Considerable weight loss, although some people eat too much and put on weight
• Gradual loss of speech
• Significant problems with short-term and long-term memory

Data from Galvin JE and Sadowsky CH. www.ncbi.nlm.nih.gov/pubmed/22570400 J Am Board Family Med. 2012;25(3):367-382.

Box 6
Alzheimer disease treatments

Current treatment approaches focus on maintaining the mental function, managing behavioral symptoms, and slowing or delaying the disease progression.

Medication: ACE inhibitors (cholinesterase inhibitors)
• Compensate for the death of cholinergic neurons. They offer symptomatic relief by inhibiting ACE turnover and restoring their synaptic levels.
• Some of the ACE inhibitor medications include donepezil, galantamine, and rivastigmine.

Self-care: creating a safe and supportive environment
• Adapting the living situation to the needs of a person with Alzheimer disease is an important part of any treatment plan.
• Always keep keys, wallets, mobile phones, and other valuables in the same place at home.
• Develop a habit of carrying a mobile phone with location capability.
• Use a calendar or whiteboard at home to track daily schedules. Build the habit of checking off completed.
• Remove excess furniture and clutter.
• Exercise regularly and eat healthy.

Data from Schneider LS. Treatment of Alzheimer's disease with cholinesterase inhibitors. Clin Geriatr Med 2001; 17:337-58.

Alzheimer disease or mixed Alzheimer disease/vascular dementia, the recommendation is combining an N-methyl-D-aspartate (NMDA) antagonist (eg, memantine) with a cholinesterase inhibitor. For moderate/severe vascular or mixed Alzheimer disease/vascular dementia, the recommendation is the control of hypertension and diabetes.

INFORMED CONSENT FOR THE COGNITIVELY IMPAIRED OLDER ADULT

Informed consent in dentistry is a patient's voluntary authorization of a dental procedure based on their understanding of the relevant information provided by the dentist. The patient's granting of informed consent for a specific treatment is the culmination of a shared decision-making process. This process is based on 1 of the 5 American Dental Association ethical principles, *autonomy*.[22,23] Assessing decision-making capacity to give informed consent typically is one of a practitioner's greatest concerns with respect to the process of shared decision making and informed consent concerning individuals with CI.

The principle for autonomy allows patients to participate in decisions regarding their treatment as well as be allowed to either consent to or refuse a proposed treatment. In cases of adults with CI, the decision making and ability to give informed consent become blurry because the dental practitioner has to assess the patient's relative cognition. In most cases, these elderly patients present to an oral health provider accompanied by a designated decision maker in the form of a health care proxy or with someone who communicates regularly and directly with the patient's decision maker. Therefore, it is crucial to obtain this information prior to the visit, and the dental office staff should be trained to seek this contact information when making the initial appointment.

Elements of Informed Consent

In cases of care for cognitively impaired persons, these conditions become even more important to consider.[24] The fact that a patient is unable to comprehend and appreciate the nature and necessity of treatment does not eliminate the necessity of informed consent.

Practitioners should ensure that they see consent as part of clinical practice rather than a barrier to providing clinical care. It is essential that the consent process is documented in the clinical records. It may require more time to gain consent from geriatric patients: however, difficulty in communicating does not mean that geriatric patients cannot give their own consent.

Five conditions are necessary to be assessed for obtaining an ethically sound informed consent[25]:

1. Patients must have capacity to make health care decisions for themselves. Sometimes the term, *competent*, is used, but this term is a legal concept and must not be misunderstood because historically an assessment of competency has strictly been made only by a court of law. Note that a person can have the capacity to make some decisions but not others; for example, a patient may have the ability to make a decision about whether or not to have root canal therapy but may not be able to make general and routine financial decisions.
2. A dentist must provide information regarding a proposed treatment as well as reasonable alternatives in a manner that allows patients (or their proxies) to become involved in treatment decisions. This information should contain (a) the nature of the proposed treatment, (b) the benefits and risks of such treatment, and (c) the benefits and risks to the alternatives to treatment, which also should include nontreatment.

3. It is not enough that patients have the ability to understand the relevant information presented; they actually must comprehend it. Many factors can interfere with a patient's comprehension, including high anxiety, fatigue, sensory deficits, and pain—symptoms that are common when dealing with the elderly population. So if individuals do not fully or substantially comprehend the relevant information, then a consent is not truly informed and thus not a valid informed consent. Because a dental care provider cannot be completely certain that a patient has sufficient understanding to make an autonomous decision, the practitioner often can make a reasonable assessment of patients' understanding by asking them to paraphrase the information presented to them.
4. The informed consent must be voluntary and without manipulation, duress, influence, or coercion because the principle of autonomy protects an individual's right to make decisions that are voluntary and intentional.
5. The informed consent is in fact the patient's authorization of a dental procedure, so patients or their proxies should be encouraged to voice their choices or put them in writing. It always is best to have the consent in writing for proper record keeping and documentation.

When a practitioner cannot assess these 5 individual elements, as in the case of a cognitively impaired elderly person, then the patient does not have the decision-making capacity about their oral health care. In this scenario, another person (proxy) becomes the surrogate decision maker; therefore, the decision-making capacity threshold passes to that person.

The best surrogate decision maker is one who knows a patient's values and preferences well. This person usually is a spouse, sibling, child, partner, or friend. Sometimes patients arrange for care decisions before losing decision-making capacity. In many instances, this is ideal, because they were of sound body and mind when they made their wishes known to their proxy. A patient may execute an advance directive in the form of a living will, which is a written document specifying what kinds of dental treatment, for example, the patient would prefer when cognitively impaired, terminally ill, or in a persistent vegetative state. Another form of advance directive is the medical power of attorney, which allows health care decisions when the patient loses decision-making capacity.[1,25]

It is integral for oral health providers to communicate the necessity of oral health to all involved parties, including the family, health care proxy, caregivers, and legal guardians. It then is highly recommended that an immediate family member or health care proxy of the aging and cognitively impaired individual becomes the supervisor of the oral health care regimens conducted by the dental caregivers.

The person who provides consent also needs to understand that in certain instances, such as with individuals with dementia, it is neither possible nor feasible to render care because doing so may endanger or have no effect on a patient's health or quality of life.[7]

The determination of providing care or no care by the health professional typically is a function of several factors, such as a thorough understanding of the patient's condition, the level of comfort and training of the health professional, and the availability of the financial resources. Many times, this decision is the greatest challenge that a treating clinician faces regarding treatment.

MULTIDISCIPLINARY APPROACH

Dental treatment of older adults living with CI may be provided in hospitals, long-term care facilities, skilled nursing facilities, private residences, group homes, private practice, or community health centers. It typically involves modifying the dental examination and the required dental treatment due to a patient's disability, impairment, and age-related conditions and symptoms.

Dental care for older patients with CI often involves consulting with 1 or more members of the patient's health care team. This effort may include but not be limited to coordinating dental treatment with other care providers, accommodating a person with the aid of the caregivers, adapting the treatment procedure, communicating through an interpreter, and customizing treatment plans with the patient's potential for future oral health problems in mind. A typical make-up of an elderly patient's health care team can include but is not limited to the following individuals:

- Dentist and dental specialist, as needed
- Primary care physician and medical specialist, as needed
- Nurse
- Nurse's aide
- Primary caregiver
- Health care proxy
- Family member(s)

The multidisciplinary team model incorporates the most effective collaborative approach in managing an older adult's health. Individuals of various health disciplines need to collaborate in developing best treatment plans and options and discuss the potential side effects or management pearls of their mutual patient because this allows team members to continuously monitor the progress actively. It also is important that all interdisciplinary team members understand the direction and goals of the dental treatment plan.

Due to the direct association between many medical conditions and the corresponding effects and problems encountered in the oral cavity, a necessary collaboration needs to be developed between the interdisciplinary team members and the dental professionals to address a patient's needs and oral manifestations appropriately[26] (Table 1). It is important that the interdisciplinary team communicate any changes in a timely manner to the group.

Oral diseases for older individuals with CI do not differ from those of older individuals without impairment.[7] Various factors related to an aging individual's disability or impairment, however, may make it more difficult to assess, prevent, and treat dental disease. For instance, someone suffering from arthritis can have difficulty grasping a toothbrush whereas someone with CI as well as arthritis may have difficulty recognizing the functionality of the toothbrush that they are having difficulty grasping. Treatment also may differ because the dental disease typically is addressed at a later stage due to infrequent check-ups, avoidance (social isolation), lack of resources, inability to articulate that a problem exists, or other common geriatric-related access-to-care issues. If this is the case, then more interdisciplinary involvement by team members typically is necessary or encouraged. Often, the care must be adapted to an individual's physical impairment and CI. Therefore, just as dental providers make adjustments to the treatment of elderly patients, it is envisioned that the dental care for those individuals with CI requires similar modifications.

Often, dental treatment of the cognitively impaired older adult can be conceptualized within 2 viewpoints simultaneously. One view is the (primary) preventive aspect of dentistry, which considers all the harmful possibilities with foresight for diseases or conditions and prophylactically applies the preventive regimens to those oral conditions so they never are manifested or, if they are, at a much lower incidence rate. The second approach is the more prevalent, therapeutic or rehabilitative aspect of

Table 1
Potential interprofessional collaboration for dental professionals

Condition	Association	Potential Collaboration with Other Health Professionals
Diabetes/A_{1C}	Evidence of routine prophylaxis reducing A_{1C} levels, improved general healing time, diabetes management	• Dieticians advising dietary controls • Primary care providers and nurses adjusting and managing medications, preventing and treating mouth infections • Pharmacists • Social workers helping with increased activities • Physical therapists and occupational therapists advising on increased activity and mobility
Loss of fine motor skills	Arthritis, stroke, neurodegenerative diseases, trauma	• Physical therapists, occupational therapists training individual to practice fine motor skills, supporting/assisting with ADLs, providing adaptive devices • Social workers coordinating transportation and payment mechanisms
Dysphagia	Stroke, Parkinson disease, Alzheimer disease, cancer treatment	• Primary care providers diagnosing condition/cause • Dietician providing guidance to prevent aspiration, recommending oral intake, diet texture
Edentulism	Compromised ability to chew, inadequate nutrition or quality of nutrition	• Primary care providers initial cancer screening • Dietician recommendation of oral intake, type and quality of nutrients, diet texture • Long-term care staff monitoring fit and function of dentures
Mucositis/glossitis	Erythematous, ulcerative lesions during cancer treatment or drug reactions	• Radiologists' and oncologists' recommendations for palliative care during therapy • Dieticians recommending avoidance of spicy, acidic, hard and hot foods and beverages • Direct care staff monitoring and providing appropriate oral hygiene products

(continued on next page)

Table 1 (continued)		
Condition	Association	Potential Collaboration with Other Health Professionals
Xerostomia	Increased susceptibility to tooth decay, swallowing difficulties. Poor selection of food products that affect glycemic control or increase carbohydrate consumption, leading to decreased quality of life due to high sugar and carbohydrate intake	• Primary care providers and nurses alerting family and patient to potential side effects, and prescribing saliva substitutes, fluoride, and other antimicrobial agents • Dieticians monitoring and advising on carbohydrate and glycemic intake • Long-term care staff monitoring the oral hygiene practices and food intake frequency and quality

Adapted from Johnson, TE, Cernohous JE, Mulhausen P, Jacobi, DA. Dental Professionals as Part of an Interdisciplinary Team, Chap 20: 268-295. Geriatric Dentistry: Caring for Our Aging Population, 2014. John Wiley & Sons, Inc.

dentistry (secondary prevention). This approach is taken once a disease or condition is encountered and typically is treated rapidly. This is the approach where we have typically spent most of our time and efforts in dentistry.[7]

The more experience gained in treating the dental needs of older adults with CI, the more it is understood that each person is different with respect to the manifestation of these conditions. In certain situations, preventive and therapeutic approaches when applied collectively can significantly improve elders' oral experience. The decision to use one approach over another, or both, is a function of patients' oral health and medical status at the time of the examination. The idea, therefore, is to illicit a model or thought process for the practitioner, where treating as well as preventing disease becomes the rule when a patient presents to a dentist. If a patient presents with no disease—an approach of "...do more now to *prevent* in order to do less treatment later..." is recommended.[7]

TREATMENT GOALS

Appropriate patient treatment goals include stabilizing and improving the oral condition of the patient. Stabilization of the oral condition keeps individuals who have not received routine oral care, have deteriorated oral health, or have received poor or inappropriate care, free of acute disease. In no way should this statement be conceived as a negative comment toward any dental team member who provided prior care for an aging individual with CI. It is reflective, however, of the common understanding and acceptance in the dental community of the need for more clinical and behavioral management training for dental team members. Often, even with the best of intentions, a dental care provider is unable to perform the best service because of lack of management skills or background knowledge on aging and disabilities for taking care of individuals with such disabilities. Treating and managing an elderly patient with CI for procedures that require multiple appointments to complete can be approached differently as long as the involved decision makers understand the modifications being proposed. For instance, replacing a failed fixed prosthesis with a new one may be addressed readily instead with a long-term, heat-cured, processed (with or without metal reinforcement) provisional at a fraction of the cost and in 1 appointment. These types of provisional restorations can be recemented, modified, relined, or repaired much more easily than frequently replacing permanent fixed bridges the conventional way.

Most of the acute oral conditions that commonly are seen in older adults as well as in individuals who have physical, cognitive, or developmental disabilities are the same as those in people who have not received adequate oral health care and present without any impairments. A clinical examination may reveal other oral conditions, however, that need appropriate or even immediate care. These conditions common in older individuals with CI are candidiasis, moniliasis, lichen planus, chronic ulcerations, fistulas, and stomatitis. With the onset of some more recent observations of osteonecrosis of the jaw due to bone cancer therapy and the use of bisphosphonates, clinicians must be even more vigilant in their clinical assessments of older adults with developmental disabilities. This is the reason why a comprehensive medical history and clinical examination cannot be overemphasized.

Once a patient is stabilized from acute disease in as many appointments as is necessary, the next phase of therapy is the restoration of the patient's teeth and missing spaces in order to address the oral health and function of the aging patient. The completion of this phase of therapy is followed by an appropriate individualized, risk-based preventative maintenance and management schedule designed to oversee a patient's re-established oral health.

MAINTENANCE MANAGEMENT

Given a patient's level of impairment or disability, the first step in obtaining compliance with oral hygiene recommendations is promoting the patient's involvement through education and demonstration. This level of involvement maximizes the patient's acceptance of their oral condition and partially promotes their independence with respect to their oral health. If a patient is unable to participate in the educational/instructional process, the caregiver is encouraged to assume this responsibility for the patient.

Educating family members or other caregivers also is critical for ensuring appropriate and regular supervision of daily oral hygiene. Caregivers should monitor a patient's oral care daily and provide oral care assistance when the patient is unable to do so. Specifically, the caregiver or family member's supervision of the aging individual with CI should include a specific routine of oral care preferably around the same time each day. This supervision may include removing any appliance(s) prior to brushing and rinsing, physically supporting or aiding the patient with routine daily tooth brushing, visually inspecting the quality of oral hygiene performance, and encouraging the individual during and after the activity. More often than not, a family member or caregiver may need to clean any appliance(s) for the patient. The most important factor, however, is making the supervised routine a daily activity.

Such supervised care can be facilitated with proper positioning of the aging patient with the aid of pillows, beanbags, airbags, and smaller/larger chairs.

Certain adaptive aids, such as large-sized toothbrush handles, may improve the manual dexterity and physical manipulation of a toothbrush. Other useful and appropriate material used in the oral health care of an aging individual with CI or physical disability may include the use of powered (rotary) toothbrushes, antimicrobial and fluoridated mouth rinses, and oral lubricants that resolve oral discomfort associated with gingival tissues and xerostomia.

Depending on where the individual with the disability resides (home, nursing home, other long-term care facility, and so forth), the primary caregiver can be a private aide, family member, nurse's aide, nurse practitioner, and/or other persons. If oral hygiene care is seen as a shared responsibility, then obtaining assistance to provide basic oral hygiene for a patient may be helpful in decreasing the level of responsibility for the primary caregiver. This could provide an additional monitoring system for a patient's oral hygiene routine as well if more individuals or aides are involved in the basic tenets of oral care for older individuals.

SUMMARY

A high degree of awareness is necessary among dental practitioners to balance the implications of a patient's CI against the demands of the dental treatment for the realistic expectation of the anticipated benefit. Dental treatment should focus on the removal of nonrestorable teeth and the maintenance of the dentition and existing dentures with frequent oral hygiene measures. In order to diminish dental pain and pathology and to maintain the dignity and quality of life of persons with CI, oral health practitioners increasingly will be involved with preserving oral and nutritional health in these patients. Dental treatment in early stages of the disease should, as far as possible, be aimed at producing a stable oral condition that gives patients minimal trouble when, in the later stages of the impairment, dental treatment may be impossible.

CLINICS CARE POINTS

- Despite the increase in MCCs with age, most people with MCCs now are individuals younger than 65 years old. This means that many more CI issues may have to be addressed in the future than currently are addressed.
- There are multiple performance-based screening tools designed for measuring cognitive issues in older adults; they include MMSE, IADL scale, ADL scale, and HAQ 8-item DI.
- ACE inhibitors currently are the most important successful treatments of Alzheimer disease. They do not stop or cure the disease, however; they only slow down or delay the progression of Alzheimer disease.
- Among nonpharmacologic interventions for mild to moderate dementia, the recommendations are caregiver education, supportive therapy, and respite care for caregivers.
- For moderate to severe Alzheimer disease or mixed Alzheimer disease/vascular dementia, the recommendation is combining an NMDA antagonist with an ACE inhibitor.
- For moderate to severe vascular or mixed Alzheimer disease/vascular dementia, the recommendation is also control of hypertension and diabetes.
- Assessing decision-making capacity to give informed consent typically is one of the practitioner's greatest concerns with respect to the process of share decision making and informed consent concerning individuals with CI.
- Five elements are necessary in obtaining an ethically sound informed consent:
  ○ Patients must have the capacity to make health care decisions for themselves.
  ○ The health care provider must provide information regarding a proposed treatment as well as reasonable alternatives in a manner that allows the patient or proxy to be involved in treatment decisions. A surrogate or proxy, therefore, is in the decision-making capacity when the patient is cognitively impaired, or the 5 elements cannot be assessed.
  ○ Patients actually must comprehend the relevant information because anxiety, fatigue, sensory deficits, and pain symptoms may interfere with comprehension.

> ○ Informed consent must be voluntary and free of manipulation.
> ○ Consent is patients' or proxies' authorization for rendering treatment, so they should be encouraged to voice their choices or put them in writing.

REFERENCES

1. Chodosh J, Petitti DB, Elliott M, et al. Physician recognition of cognitive impairment: evaluating the need for improvement. J Am Geriatr Soc 2004;52(7):1051–9.
2. Albert MS, DeKosky ST, Dickson D, et al. The diagnosis of mild cognitive impairment due to Alzheimer's disease: recommendations from the National Institute on Aging-Alzheimer's Association workgroups on diagnostic guidelines for Alzheimer's disease. Alzheimers Dement 2011;7(3):270–9.
3. U.S Census Bureau. Available at: www.census.gov. Accessed May 29, 2020.
4. Adams ML. Differences between younger and older US adults with multiple chronic conditions. Prev Chronic Dis 2017;14:E76.
5. Holsinger T, Deveau J, Boustani M, et al. Does this patient have dementia? JAMA 2007;297(21):2391–404.
6. McCarten JR. Clinical evaluation of early cognitive symptoms. Clin Geriatr Med 2013;29(4):791–807.
7. Farsai P, Calabrese J. Treatment Considerations: Specific to the Aging Population with Disabilities (4) 83-96. Treating the Dental Patient with Developmental Disorder Wiley-Blackwell 2012.
8. Cornelis E, Gorus E, Van Schelvergem N, et al. The relationship between basic, instrumental, and advanced activities of daily living and executive functioning in geriatric patients with neurocognitive disorders. Int J Geriatr Psychiatry 2019; 34(6):889-899.
9. Truhlar MR. Geriatric patient Assessment, Chap 6: 61-69. Geriatric dentistry: caring for our aging population. New York: John Wiley & Sons, Inc; 2014.
10. Soleimani R, Shokrgozar S, Fallahi M, et al. Correction to: An investigation into the prevalence of cognitive impairment and the performance of older adults in Guilan province. J Med Life 2018;11(4):395.
11. Barnes DE, Beiser AS, Lee A, et al. Development and validation of a brief dementia screening indicator for primary care. Alzheimers Dement 2014;10(6): 656–65.e1.
12. Harper KJ, Riley V, Jacques A, et al. Australian modified Lawton's Instrumental Activities of Daily Living Scale contributes to diagnosing older adults with cognitive impairment. Australas J Ageing 2019;38(3):199–205.
13. McPherson S, Schoephoester G. Screening for dementia in a primary care practice. Minn Med 2012 Jan;95(1):36–40.
14. Bradford A, Kunik M, Schulz P, et al. Missed and delayed diagnosis of dementia in primary care: prevalence and contributing factors. Alzheimer Dis Assoc Disord 2009;23(4):306–13.
15. Boustani M, Peterson B, Hanson L, et al. Screening for dementia in primary care: a summary of the evidence for the U.S. Preventive Services Task Force. Ann Intern Med 2003;138(11):927–37.
16. Kotagal V, Langa KM, Plassman BL, et al. Factors associated with cognitive evaluations in the United States. Neurology 2014;84(1):64–71.
17. Sanford AM. Mild Cognitive Impairment. Clin Geriatr Med 2017;33(3):325–37.
18. Hugo J, Ganguli M. Dementia and cognitive impairment: epidemiology, diagnosis, and treatment. Clin Geriatr Med 2014;30(3):421–42.

19. Gao Y, Tan L, Yu JT, et al. Tau in Alzheimer's disease: mechanisms and therapeutic strategies. Curr Alzheimer Res 2018;15(3):283–300.
20. Schneider LS. Treatment of Alzheimer's disease with cholinesterase inhibitors. Clin Geriatr Med 2001;17:337–58.
21. Kocaelli H, Yaltirik M, Yargic LI, et al. Alzheimer's disease and dental management. Oral Surg Oral Med Oral Pathol Oral Radiol Endod 2002;93(5):521–4.
22. Lo B. Assessing decision-making capacity. Law Med Health Care 1990;18:193.
23. Wettle T. Ethical issues in geriatric dentistry. Gerodontology 1987;6:73.
24. Mukherjee A, Livinski AA, Millum J, et al. Informed consent in dental care and research for the older adult population: A systematic review. J Am Dent Assoc 2017;148(4):211–20.
25. Annas GJ. The health care proxy and the living will. N Engl J Med 1991;324:1210.
26. Johnson TE, Cernohous JE, Mulhausen P, et al. Dental professionals as part of an interdisciplinary team, Chap 20: 268-295. Geriatric dentistry: caring for our aging population. New York: John Wiley & Sons, Inc; 2014.

Consideration in Planning Dental Treatment of Older Adults

Ronald Ettinger, MDS, DDSc, DDSc(hc)[a],
Leonardo Marchini, DDS, MSD, PhD[b],*, Jennifer Hartshorn, DDS[c]

KEYWORDS

• Aged • Frail elderly • Mental health • Root caries • Oral health • Oral hygiene

KEY POINTS

- Frail and functionally dependent older adults include a diverse group of people with multiple disabilities, which are influenced further by their life experiences that complicate decisions related to clinical dental care.
- Furthermore, because they grew up prior to water fluoridation, most of them have maintained some of their teeth, but this puts them at higher risk for coronal and root caries, which complicates restorative care.
- The decision-making process, which has evolved, essentially has developed into a treatment planning philosophy that takes into account the best interests of the patient after evaluating all the modifying factors.

INTRODUCTION

In 2020, the total US population was approximately 330 million person and those aged 65 years and older made up nearly 16%, which is approximately 53 million persons.[1] There is greater heterogeneity among people aged 65 years and older than in any other age group.[2] Each older adult has a unique genome and has been influenced by a variety of environmental factors, such as social, cultural, economic, and cohort experiences, that have determined their lifestyle and health beliefs.[3] The oral health of these individuals also is affected by these same factors, so, when planning dental

This article originally appeared in Dental Clinics, Volume 65 Issue 2, April 2021.
[a] Department of Prosthodontics, The University of Iowa College of Dentistry and Dental Clinics, N-409 Dental Science, Iowa City, IA 52242, USA; [b] Department of Preventive and Community Dentistry, The University of Iowa College of Dentistry and Dental Clinics, N337-1 Dental Science, Iowa City, IA 52242, USA; [c] Department of Preventive and Community Dentistry, The University of Iowa College of Dentistry and Dental Clinics, W327 Dental Science, Iowa City, IA 52242, USA
* Corresponding author.
E-mail address: leonardo-marchini@uiowa.edu

treatment of older adults, dentists must take into account the social aspects, general health, and oral health conditions prior to delivering care.[4]

In geriatric medicine, it is important to make a diagnosis, and, once a diagnosis is made, there usually is enough scientific evidence to support a treatment plan. In geriatric dental medicine, it also is important to make a diagnosis, but often there are multiple treatment strategies, which often are not evidence based. Also, dentistry is unlike internal medicine and more like surgery, in that dentists need to remove infected tissue and restore shape and function, which require operating equipment.[5]

Therefore, if an older adult can drive or use public transport independently to access a dental office, this removes a significant complication associated with their treatment.[6] These persons have been defined as functionally independent older adults and comprise approximately 70% of persons over the age of 65 years. In general, they live in the community without assistance, but many may have 1 or more chronic medical problems, such as hypertension, type 2 diabetes mellitus, osteoarthritis, and so forth, for which they are taking a variety of medications.[3] To treat these older adults, dentists must take a thorough medical and drug history and understand how these diseases and medications influence patients' oral health conditions and dental treatment. The treatment such patients accept depends on their own and their significant others'/family members' perceptions of need for care as well as the amount of money they are prepared to spend on that care.[5]

A smaller group of older adults (approximately 20%) can be designated as frail older adults, because they have lost some of their independence.[3] They still are living in the community with the help of family and friends and may be using professional support services, such as Meals on Wheels, home health aides, visiting nurses, and so forth.[3] These frail older adults can access dental services only with the help of others if they are provided with transport. To treat this population, the dentist needs a greater knowledge of medicine and pharmacology as well as the skill to evaluate a patient's ability to maintain daily oral hygiene independently. Another important factor is the patient's ability to tolerate the treatment that has been proposed.[5]

The smallest group of older adults (approximately 10%) have been called functionally dependent older adults.[3] These persons are unable to survive in the community independently and either are homebound (5%) or living in a long-term care institution (5%). A minority of these older adults can be transported to a dental office provided it is wheelchair accessible, and a dentist is willing to care for them. The majority need to be cared for at their home or in their institution. To care for them, the dental professionals need either mobile dental equipment or a dental office in the long-term care facility.[5]

TREATMENT PLANNING
Patient Interview

The initial contact between older adults and their dentist begins with telephone contact between the patient/caregiver and the dental office receptionist. Therefore, a receptionist needs to have been sensitized to eliciting important information from potential patients, especially if they are frail or functionally dependent. To treat these patients safely, there is a need to know whether a patient needs help with transportation,[7,8] any specific accommodations for wheelchairs or oxygen tanks, the availability to come for an appointment, the chief complaint,[9] and current health issues,[9] including questions about symptoms of 2019 Coronvirus Disease (COVID-19).[10] The receptionist also ask the should patients/caregivers to bring a list of current medications or the medications themselves[5,9]; a list of their health care providers; and dental radiographs if they exist. The receptionist needs to be empathetic to the age-associated sensory deficits of the patient, which can result in longer conversations to acquire the desired information and to schedule appointments.[11]

Teledentistry

The COVID-19 pandemic has thrust teledentistry to the forefront of dental practices. Teledentistry may be beneficial particularly for those who are considered at high risk of severe illness or mortality associated with COVID-19 infection, because efforts are being made to minimize Severe Acute Respiratory Syndrome Coronovirus 2 transmission to this vulnerable population. The use of teledentistry, however, will transcend this pandemic as a useful tool for dentists, the public, and especially at-risk populations. This vulnerable population includes but is not limited to persons of any age with multiple comorbidities, those over age 65 years, persons who are immunocompromised, and those residing in nursing homes.[10] A national survey has reported that older adults in the United States are interested in utilizing teledentistry but have expressed some concern with managing the technology needed to access virtual appointments.[12] Teledentistry is particularly useful, however, in evaluating nursing home patients because it allows the dentist and the nursing facility resident to remain in their respective locations while nursing home staff manage the technology needed to complete the visit.[13] Although these residents still may need an in-person dental appointment, the information gathered during these teledentistry visits can reduce the time in the dental office waiting room in order to complete forms and preappointment consent from the resident and/or person with power of attorney and, therefore, expedite treatment that minimizes the at-risk person's exposure time to the public. Teledentistry similarly can be advantageous for older adults living at home, but efforts should be made to select a simple technology that is easily accessible and overcomes any sensory deficits, such as hearing loss, either via synchronous (live video) or asynchronous (forwarding a still photo to the dentist) methods. Instances in which dentists will find teledentistry immediately helpful is when triaging a new or existing older adult patient prior to entering the dental clinic, diagnosing and treatment planning for existing dental patients, and postprocedural management of those patients.[14]

As patients come for the initial appointments, usually they are handed multiple forms about patient registration, finances, and health history. It is assumed that patients are literate, cognitively not impaired, and can understand the information being sought. The National Adult Literacy Survey reported, however, that 59% of the US older adult population had basic or below proficiency in health literacy, which means they would have difficult interpreting health-related printed materials.[15] Patients' age-associated impaired vision and slower cognitive processing of information exacerbate the problem of understanding printed materials, which often can slow the usual pace of a dental office.[15]

Consequently, when interviewing an older adult patient, the dentist should use the completed forms to begin the conversation with the patient/caregiver but extend the interview to include an evaluation of all the potential modifying factors. Good communication with patients and their significant others requires investigative interviewing when assessing patients with complex social and medical/mental conditions, in order to understand the hidden meanings of their complaints.[5] If dentists are not sensitized to understand the true nature of the implications of the chief complaint, they may miss important clues. For instance, a 72-year-old patient from a practice returns because she has lost the crown on her central incisor. Previously, she had returned for routine care regularly every 6 months, but she has been missing her appointments for more than 2 years. On careful questioning, she reported that 2 years ago her husband died unexpectedly, and her children live in distant states. Her health and overall grooming have deteriorated visibly as has her oral hygiene. It is clear that she is suffering from severe depression associated with sustained grief due to the loss of her husband and her own health and mobility. She urgently needs counseling and mental health care. Merely treating her current dental problems does not address her essential needs. Therefore, focusing only on her current dental problem can lead to continuous oral deterioration or even more life-threatening consequences.

In assessing patient health histories, it is important to interpret the information provided by careful questioning. For example, if a patient reports a has a history of angina pectoris, what does this really mean? Does the patient experience spontaneous chest pain or by walking from the car to the office or by going up a set of stairs, or did the patient have chest pain 6 months ago and no episodes since then? Each of these scenarios requires the dentist to modify the management of the patient, due to the risk of precipitating potential medical problems. Possible modifications might range from using a stress-reducing protocol to postponing elective treatment until patients have been assessed by their physician.

HOW DO DENTISTS MAKE DECISIONS?

When examining how dentists make decisions, it should be that considered a majority of oral diseases are chronic plaque-associated diseases, such as caries and periodontal disease, which cause irreversible damage.[16] Some diseases of the oral mucosa and pulp can be cured, whereas a few, such as oral neoplasms, are life-threatening.[5,16] A majority of oral health needs in older adults are treating the exacerbations of caries and periodontal disease.[5,17,18]

Clinical geriatric dentistry requires problem solving and decision making to develop an appropriate treatment plan. In younger adults, the factors that influence the decision making related to treatment planning are simpler; for instance, Does the patient have the will and the time to accept the care? Does the patient wish to pay for the care? and Does the dentist have the resources and skills to carry out that care? In older adults, the factors may become more complex, and the dentist needs more skills and experience in decision making to develop an age-appropriate treatment plan. This treatment plan should take into account the multiplicity of modifying factors, which include but are not limited to patient's socioeconomic, psychological, and medical problems; side-effects of their medications; and the cumulative effects of dental diseases as well as the iatrogenic effects on the dentition due to previous dental care.[19,20]

The knowledge base to manage the treatment planning process for older adults does not require the development of new technical skills but rather the development of thought processes to understand the patient's modifying factors and how they may influence treatment. The aim of treatment is to understand how patients are functioning in their environment and how their dental needs and treatment fit into their lifestyle. When making these decisions, the benefits of treatment must outweigh the risks of adverse events. The thought processes that are required to develop this treatment protocol were developed by Ettinger and Beck,[21] and have been called, "rational treatment planning."

To make these decisions requires the gathering of information from and about the patient, in order to be able to make a diagnosis and a treatment plan. There have been several systems suggested in the literature on how to gather and process this information.[5] One of the most used systems is a modification of the American Society of Anesthesiologists evaluation scheme to assess patients' ability to tolerate treatment. This system has been used as a reference to modify therapy and patient management and provides guidelines for the dental treatment of medically compromised patients, especially those who need anesthesia.[22] This system was modified by Kamen[23] into 4 broad categories (**Fig. 1**). Gordon and Kress[24] identified some of the faults of this system by stating, "when applied to specific situations, the system is somewhat simplistic, in that many patients fall between categories and many choices remain even within one category."

Another such system uses the mnemonic, subjective findings, objective findings, assessment, and plan (SOAP).[25] For older adults, subjective findings must include information on functional status, such as activities of daily living (ADLs) and instrumental activities of daily living (IADLs). Objective findings include an oral examination, radiographs, and other intraoral and laboratory findings. Using these findings leads a dentist to an assessment of the patient's expectations and needs, which evolves into a treatment plan.

Shay[26] has proposed another mnemonic, which he called OSCAR, especially designed for older adults. The O stands for oral factors, the S for systemic factors, the C for capability, the A for autonomy, and the R for reality. The oral factors include the condition of the dentition, restorations, periodontium, coronal and root caries, tooth loss, salivary function, mucosal health, oral hygiene, and the occlusion. Systemic factors should include an assessment of general health, available laboratory findings, the impact of medications, and communication between the dentist and the patient's physicians. Capability addresses the patients ADLs and IADLs as well as issues, such as incontinence. Autonomy relates primarily to a patient's ability to provide informed consent independently and maintain oral hygiene, which might be impaired as a result of stroke, dementia, or other diseases that affect cognitive function. Reality takes into account life expectancy and a patient's ability to access care and pay for the required treatment.

A similar but somewhat different conceptual model was suggested by Berkey and colleagues.[27] They proposed that decision making for older adults requires clinicians to take into account 4 domains, which are function, symptomatology, pathology, and

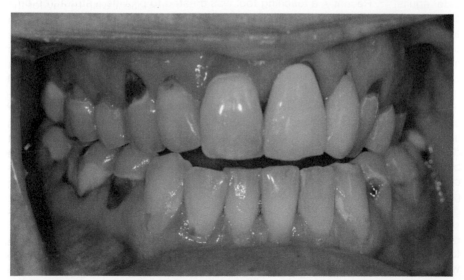

Fig. 1. Full mouth view of Mrs LL's dentition, showing multiple root caries lesions as well as generalized gingival recession. Plaque levels are limited to the lower one-third of the teeth, with relatively little gingival inflammation.

esthetics. Function relates to the ability of the patient to chew and eat an adequate diet. Symptomatology assesses the amount of pain or discomfort when chewing and having adequate amounts of saliva to speak, to taste and to swallow. Pathology evaluates oral discomfort and the presence of lesions in the mouth. Esthetics focuses on the patients' expectations to improve their appearance or smile. In order to achieve these assessments, the investigators[27] suggested that clinicians need to ask older adults the following questions:

1. What are the patient's desires and expectations with regard to dental treatment?
2. What are the type and severity of dental needs?
3. What is the impact of dental treatment on quality of life?
4. What is the probability of positive outcomes of dental treatment?
5. What are reasonable dental treatment alternatives?
6. What is the ability of the patient to tolerate the stress of dental treatment?
7. What is the capability of the patient to maintain oral health?
8. What are the patient's financial and other resources to pay for dental treatment?
9. What is the dentist's capability of achieving the planned dental treatment?
10. Are there any other issues?

Using the answers to these questions, the dentist then could determine what level of care was achievable for the patient, which could be very extensive care, extensive care, intermediate care, limited care, or very limited care. Very extensive care includes complex rehabilitation, such as fixed prosthodontics and implants. Extensive care may be a combination of fixed and removable prosthodontics. Intermediate care requires a modification of traditional therapies, such as an interim prosthesis. Limited care suggests that patients cannot tolerate extensive treatment time in the dental chair and require short appointments and simplified treatment. Very limited care focuses only on pain relief and infection control.

Various other models have been proposed to aid the clinician in decision making, especially with regard to the medically at risk and frail and functionally dependent older adults[9,28]. Recently, a teaching tool was created to provide a structured process to guide novice students when caring for frail and functionally dependent older adults. This teaching tool helps the students to process the overwhelming amount of information gathered from their patients and helps them to develop a decision-making process that would lead them to rational treatment planning. This concept, which has been called rapid oral health deterioration (ROHD) risk assessment, also may be useful for the practicing dentist.[4]

The concept was developed because more older adults are keeping their teeth into older age, which has complicated dental treatment.[29] There is evidence that as they age the risk of oral disease, which negatively affects their dentition or results in the deterioration of their general health, increases.[18] ROHD has been based on evidence based risk factors, which have been classified into 3 categories: (1) general health conditions, (2) social support, and (3) oral health conditions. Briefly, in the first category, there are multiple diseases, which influence a patient's ability to maintain oral hygiene, which would increase their risk of ROHD. Some of the concepts included in the social support category are lack of income or dental insurance, dependency on caregivers, transportation barriers, being institutionalized or homebound, and being able to access adequate nutrition as well as having had the benefit of lifelong community water fluoridation. The oral condition category encompasses factors, such as dry mouth and xerostomia associated with disease and polypharmacy, lesions of the oral mucosa, level of oral hygiene, number of heavily restored teeth, amount of coronal and root caries, degree of periodontal disease, and presence of fixed and removable prosthesis.[4] **Box 1** presents the detailed steps used for treatment planning based on the concepts of ROHD risk assessment.

RATIONAL TREATMENT PLANNING

After gathering and processing the data from the clinical assessment of the patient, the dentist needs to develop viable treatment alternatives that are compatible with a patient's lifestyle and modifying factors. The rational treatment planning philosophy can guide the development of these treatment alternatives, by using evidence-based data, where available, to make decisions.[21]

Caries is prevalent among frail and functionally dependent older adults who have teeth that have been treated and retreated over the years,[14] which makes restoring this dentition complex. Rational treatment planning evaluates the modifying factors to offer a realistic treatment plan that has the best potential outcome for the patient. For instance, the tooth may need to be extracted, the recurrent caries could be excavated and the existing restoration repaired with a glass ionomer, the whole restoration may need to be replaced, or the tooth may need to be crowned. The decision would depend on the patient's access to care, the systemic health of the patient, the extent of the carious lesion, and patient's ability to tolerate treatment and to maintain oral hygiene as well as ability to pay for care. A principle that could guide the decision is minimally invasive dentistry (MID), which contends that caries is a chronic infectious disease and should be treated using a medical model rather than a mechanistic one. The primary components of MID are assessment of the risk of disease, with a focus on early detection and preservation of dental tissue, external and internal remineralization, and using a range of materials with surgical intervention only when the disease has been controlled.[30,31]

Box 1
Steps in treatment planning using the rapid oral health deterioration assessment

Step 1. Gathering information concerning ROHD risk factors
a. General health conditions
b. Social support
c. Oral health conditions

Step 2. Prioritizing the information and developing an appropriate communication plan
a. What matter most for disease progression and treatment planning?
b. What will happen if the patient does not receive dental care?
c. An appropriate communication plan includes but is not limited to explaining the findings, the prognosis, the treatment alternatives, and the maintenance plan to the patient and care personnel.

Step 3. Categorizing the risk for ROHD
a. Risk factors are not present; therefore, ROHD is not occurring.
b. Risk factors are present; however, ROHD currently is not occurring.
c. Risk factors are present, and ROHD currently is occurring.
d. Risk factors are present, and ROHD already has occurred.

Step 4. Identifying possible treatment alternatives compatible with rational treatment planning
a. Comprehensive care
b. Limited care (maintenance and monitoring)
c. Emergency care (pain and infection control)
d. No treatment

Step 5. Developing a maintenance plan

Some of the alternatives to the treatment of caries in frail and functionally dependent older adults, especially those with severe cognitive impairment, that derive from MID is the use of silver diamine fluoride (SDF) only to arrest caries.[32] If the patient is relatively uncooperative, then atraumatic restorative technique can be used to hand excavate the caries and restore the tooth with a glass ionomer.[33,34] Less cognitively impaired patients may tolerate the use of more traditional restorative techniques. Topical application of fluoride varnish on a regular basis is recommended for all patients.[35]

Although edentulism has declined, tooth loss still is a major oral health problem, especially among older adults.[29] Evidence-based guidelines to replace a missing tooth are virtually nonexistent.[5] Answering the problem, however, requires evaluating patients' dentition and determining several factors,[5] such as

1. How long has the tooth been missing? If the extractions are recent, then it is important to look at the occluding pairs of teeth, which determines the stability of the occlusion.
2. Is the extracted tooth an antagonist and has it moved? If there is an antagonist and if the extraction is recent, then a replacement may be necessary to preserve the occlusal plane.
3. Is there an esthetic problem? If the missing tooth is in the anterior of the mouth and the patient is severely cognitively impaired, replacement of that tooth with a prosthesis needs to be evaluated carefully. The decision requires a discussion with patients and person with power of attorney in terms of the risk of a prosthesis increasing plaque retention as well as on the preservation of the rest of the dentition.
4. Can the patient chew comfortably and effectively? Are there adequate numbers of occluding pairs of teeth, as suggested by Käyser.[36]
5. Is there any temporomandibular joint pain? If patients report temporomandibular dysfunction pain, they may need posterior support of the occlusion provided by a prosthesis.

When considering replacing posterior missing teeth, it should be kept in mind the concept of the shortened dental arch introduced by the studies of Käyser,[36] who showed that patients had sufficient adaptive capacity to maintain adequate oral function if they had at least 4 posterior occlusal units remaining, preferably in a symmetric position. They have been several studies that have supported the shortened dental arch concept, functionally,[37] financially,[38] and as it relates to quality of life.[39]

The maintenance of remaining teeth in older adults becomes important, especially for older adults with a variety of systemic diseases. Persons with neurodegenerative diseases, such as Parkinson disease, tardive dyskinesia, stroke, and dementia, are unable to adapt to complete dentures, especially on the mandibular arch. Therefore, the maintenance of some mandibular teeth is critical to maintain adequate oral function. Some of these teeth become more valuable than others, and these teeth have been described as key teeth (**Box 2**).

The available options for dental treatment have increased dramatically over time. As the total number of dental journals indexed by *Journal Citation Reports* available on the Institute for Scientific Information Web of Knowledge database has increased from 46 in 2003 to 83 in 2012, in the same time period, the number of publications in dental journals more than doubled, from 4727 to 10,102.[40] This number of publications is equivalent to more than 27 articles per day. These options include new restorative and preventive materials as well as new techniques, such as implants and digital dentistry. Treatment planning, however, still remains as much as art as science.

> **Box 2**
> **Characteristics of key teeth**
>
> A key tooth
> 1. Is one that can support itself or other teeth
> 2. Is one, which, if lost dramatically, changes the treatment plan, such as
>   • From no prosthesis to a fixed partial denture
>   • From a fixed partial denture to a removable partial denture
>   • From a tooth supported partial denture to a distal extension removable partial denture
>   • From a removable partial denture to an overdenture/complete denture
> 3. Is one that is required to maintain an adequate chewing pair

MRS LL CASE

For example, the authors were contacted by the director of nursing from a local nursing home about a 77-year-old woman (Mrs LL), who was avoiding certain foods. The patient had not seen a dentist in at least 2 years, and the staff were concerned that she might have some "dental problems." An appointment was arranged for the patient, who was wheelchair bound. Transportation and an escort were provided by the nursing home, who brought the patient's medical record and a list of her medication. The record showed that Mrs LL's son lived in a distant state and had power of attorney, but visited his mother several times a year. On contacting her son for permission to examine Mrs LL, he told the authors that he was financially responsible for her dental care. The escort told the authors that Mrs LL loves ice cream but recently has refused to eat it.

Medical History

The patient is allergic to dimenhydrinate (Dramamine). She has a history of hypothyroidism that was diagnosed 10 years ago, history of Parkinson disease with mild tremors (3 years ago), history of gastroesophageal reflux (3 years ago), dementia (2 years ago), depression (2 years ago), and insomnia (10 years ago). She also has chronic pain and muscle weakness.

Daily Medications

Mrs LL was taking multiple medications for her illnesses, many of which had significant systemic and oral side effects, as shown in **Table 1**.

Oral Health Findings

The patient was not concerned about esthetics; although she did not complain about any discomfort, the staff told the authors that she always loved ice cream and recently was avoiding it. On oral examination, Mrs LL is fully dentate, except for third molars and first premolars, which had been extracted for orthodontic purposes. A majority of teeth were covered with plaque at the gingival margins; however, there was little evidence of inflammation and no significant pocket depths. There was gingival recession and root surface caries on multiple teeth in both arches (see **Fig. 1**). The radiographic evaluation showed some bone loss in the mandibular anterior region. There was evidence of root canal treatments on teeth #9 and #10, with no visible periapical radiolucencies (**Fig. 2**). Although the patient did not complain of a dry mouth and the clinical examination did not suggest a lack of moisture, multiple root surface lesions suggest that there may be a change in the quality of the saliva. Mrs LL was able to follow directions, was able to cooperate during the oral examination, and had minimal tremors of the head and neck.

Table 1
Daily medications

Drug	Dosage	Commercial/Generic Name	Use	Side Effects
Bisacodyl	5 mg qd	Dulcolax	Laxative	Gastrointestinal discomfort, cramps, semi-supine chair position
Diphenhydramine	25 mg q6h	Benadryl	Antihistamine	Somnolence, dizziness, hypotension, sedation, dry mouth, nose and throat
Guaifenesin	2 mg q4h	Robitussin	Expectorant	Dizziness, headache, nausea, gastrointestinal pain
Hydrocodone/Acettaminophen	5 mg q6h	Vicodin	Opioid analgesic	Dizziness, sedation, bradycardia, risk of psychological and physiologic dependence, orthostatic hypotension
Levothyroxine	50 µg qd	Synthroid	Thyroid hormone	Hair loss, dry skin
Loperamide	2 mg qd (prn)	Imodium	Antidiarrheal opioid	Dry mouth, somnolence, semi-supine position
Miconazole	200 mg bid	Monistat-Derm	Imidazole antifungal	Rash, itching, dizziness, can increase bleeding with warfarin
MiraLAX	17 g qd	Polyethylene glycol 3350	Laxative	Bloating, dizziness, blood in the stool
Mirtazapine	7.5 mg hs	Remeron	Tetracyclic antidepressant	Somnolence, dry mouth, constipation, weight gain. dizziness, semi-supine position
Nystatin ointment	1000 U 4×/day	Mycostatin	Fungistatic antifungal	Rash
Omeprazole	20 mg qd	Prilosec	Proton pump inhibitor	Headache; nausea, cough, dry mouth
Quetiapine	25 mg bid	Seroquel	Antipsychotic	Headache, somnolence, dizziness, dry mouth, constipation, tachycardia, orthostatic hypotension, tardive dyskinesia, frequent recalls
Risperidone	2 mg bid	Risperdal	Antipsychotic	Agitation, anxiety, insomnia, constipation, rhinitis, orthostatic hypotension, dry mouth, extrapyramidal movements, limit vasoconstrictors, semi-supine position
Sinemet	0.5 mg bid	Carbidopa/levodopa	Antiparkinsonian	Uncontrolled body movements, nausea, anorexia, depression, anxiety, confusion, dry mouth, orthostatic hypotension, photophobia (dark glasses)
Trazadone	25 mg hs	Desyrel	Antidepressant	Somnolence, dizziness, nausea, blurred vision, light headache, orthostatic hypotension, dry mouth
Tylenol	650 mg q6h	Acetaminophen	Nonnarcotic analgesic	Hypersensitivity, liver damage with dosage of 3000 mg/d

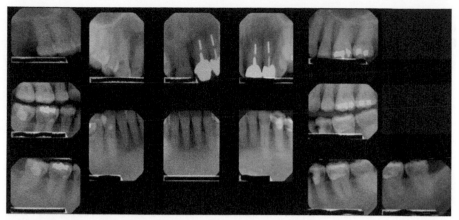

Fig. 2. Full mouth radiographs, including bitewing radiographs made at the initial appointment, showing multiple caries lesions and root canal treatment of teeth #9 and #10.

After examining the patient and gathering data (**Box 3**), the question was how should Mrs LL's oral health needs be approached? One approach would be to prioritize the risk factors that are more important for disease progression and treatment planning (see **Box 3**). When evaluating medical and social history, the impact of her developing dementia and Parkinson disease suggests that she will need increasing help with her daily oral hygiene over time and dietary changes to reduce her sugar intake. An electric toothbrush has been shown to be beneficial in this population, provided patients can tolerate it.[41] Additional preventive measures will be needed, such as the use of topical fluoride varnish, a prescription for high-concentration daily fluoride toothpaste, and a return dental visit every 3 months.[42]

If the necessary preventive measures and treatment are not accepted, there will be further progression of root surface caries, with fracture of the teeth with possible local pain and infection, resulting in periapical lesions and loss of function. Consequently, there could be a possible deterioration of Mrs LL's systemic health and quality of life and the potential for aspiration pneumonia, which can be life threatening. Therefore, Mrs LL is presenting with multiple ROHD risk factors, and ROHD currently is occurring (see **Box 3**).

Box 3
Modified American Society of Anesthesiologists classification for frail and functionally dependent older adults[23]

Class I. Comprehensive dental treatment, including all necessary surgical, operative, prosthetic, and preventive services

Class II. Intermediate dental care, emphasizing preservation and maintenance of the existing dentition and prevention of further deterioration. This can range from restorative dentistry to a simple prophylaxis.

Class III. Emergency dental care only. This includes alleviation of pain, infection, and/or swelling. This is palliative care, applicable even for terminally ill patients.

Class IV. No dental treatment, a decision based on physical and mental contraindications for care, when treatment would do more harm than good.

Considering the extensiveness of the current caries lesions and the patient's ability to cooperate, it is possible to choose multiple options to treat Mrs LL's dentition (see **Box 3**). For instance,

1. Comprehensive care, such as excavating the lesions to determine their depth. If they are shallow, complete caries removal is possible. If a lesion is deep, then partial caries removal should be considered, with glass ionomer applied to the deepest areas. The use of a sandwich technique may be appropriate, or, if the lesion is very large or very deep, it may be necessary to do a root canal treatment and/or to crown the tooth.
3. Limited care might include
   a. The use of atraumatic restorative technique to hand excavate the lesions and restore with glass ionomer, associated with home preventive measures and 6 month recalls
   b. The use of SDF to arrest the carious lesions and 6-month recalls with SDF reapplication
   c. The use of fluoride varnish in the office followed by the daily use of high-concentration fluoride toothpaste and recalls every 3 months
3. Emergency care (pain and infection control)

Emergency care may be the first step in a comprehensive care plan, or it could be the choice of a patient who seeks only comfort for the problem. If the patient presents with odontogenic pain or a dental abscess, however, it is important to define the source and treat the offending tooth or extract it. It may be necessary to support this treatment with oral antibiotics. If the pain is from a nonodontogenic source, then it is important to define the cause and treat the problem appropriately. It may be necessary to refer the patient to an appropriate medical or dental specialist for care.

4. No treatment.

If a patient seeks a consultation, is offered a treatment plan, and refuses treatment, the dentist needs to document this encounter in detail. If patients are so impaired that they cannot tolerate transfer to a dental office or any procedure in their mouth, however, a caretaker may help to reduce the bacterial burden by spraying chlorhexidine in the mouth on a daily basis.[43]

Box 4
Classification of patients with chronic unstable medical problems

Type I
  Patients with chronic existing problem(s), for example, post–cerebrovascular accident, asthma, chronic bronchitis, coronary artery disease
  These diseases progress but usually at a slow rate.
  Time is *not* a problem, because treatment can be phased in a little at a time to keep stress low.

Type II
  Patients with progressive medical problem(s), for example, dementia, cardiomyopathy, myasthenia gravis, scleroderma
  These diseases progress at a relatively faster rate, and patients deteriorate with time:
  • Need to maintain and preserve key teeth
  • Need to remove questionable teeth
  • If necessary, need to crown teeth
  Time is a problem, because patients need to be treated while they are able to tolerate treatment.

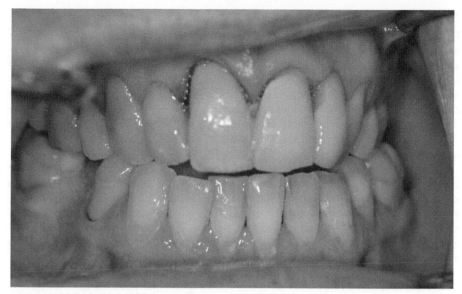

Fig. 3. Full mouth view of Mrs LL's dentition, showing the completed glass ionomer restorations. Tooth #30 has been extracted, because it was deemed unrestorable.

At this point, Mrs LL's son was contacted to inform him of his mother's oral health status and her treatment needs. In order to get informed consent (either verbally or in a signed document) to allow the authors to treat Mrs LL, the authors informed him about the different treatment options and their costs and suggested a rational treatment plan. This rational treatment plan included an evaluation of Mrs LL's cognitive status and ability to cooperate with the amount of dental treatment she needed as well as the authors' ability to deliver this care. An assessment of her chronic medical problems will help determine the need for phasing of her treatment, as shown in **Box 4**. Another important consideration was the nursing home staff's ability and willingness to commit to carry out daily oral hygiene in order to keep the appropriate maintenance regimen.

The treatment plan suggested and that her son accepted was as follows:

1. Scaling, cleaning, and polishing with fluoride varnish application, followed by customized oral hygiene instructions, including information for the nursing staff on how to maintain Mrs LL's daily care
2. A prescription for 5000 parts per million fluoride toothpaste, which should be sodium lauryl sulfate–free
3. Systematic restoration of the carious lesions using incomplete caries removal to determine restorability
     In the maxilla: from teeth #2 to #4, #6 to #11, and #13 to #15: cervical glass ionomer restorations
     In the mandible: from teeth #18 to #20, #23 and #27, #29 and #31: cervical glass ionomer restorations. Tooth #22 was deemed to be able to be remineralized with topical application of fluoride varnish
     Teeth #24 to #26 did not require any restorations.
     Tooth #30 was deemed unrestorable and was extracted.
     The completed dental treatment of Mrs LL after 4 weeks is shown in **Fig. 3**.
4. Patient was put on 3-months' recall and has returned consistently for the past 2 years, and recurrent caries occurred on tooth #14.

SUMMARY

The case of Mrs LL history presented illustrates the significant changes that have occurred in the aging population, that is, the maintenance of a natural dentition into old age. It also illustrates the problems and risks this presents for the patient and those who care for them. The chronic medical problems of the patient, especially the dementia and Parkinson disease, which are progressive diseases, will cause limitations in the patient's ability to cooperate and follow instructions over time and put this patient's oral health at risk. Therefore, it was important to involve the family (son) and the care staff at the nursing home in the patient's restorative care as well as in the maintenance of her oral health.

In addition, modern restorative techniques need to be used, such as minimal invasive dentistry, including incomplete caries removal and sealing the lesions with glass ionomer, followed by a high concentration of topical fluoride to prevent further demineralization. The treatment followed the overall ethical principles, which are to do no harm and to do treatment that benefits the patient. This treatment was well tolerated and should improve the quality of her life (eg, allow her to enjoy her ice cream) and maintain function.

It is the authors' belief that the successful treatment of frail and functionally dependent older adults must include an understanding of how patients are functioning (medically, socially, and emotionally) in their environment and how the art and science of dental medicine fit into that environment.

CLINICS CARE POINTS

- Teledentistry should be considered when triaging new or existing older adult patients prior to their entering the dental clinic. Teledentistry also can be used for diagnosing and treatment planning for an existing dental patient as well as for postprocedural management.

- Good communication with patients and their significant others requires investigative interviewing when assessing patients with complex social and medical/mental conditions.

- In assessing patients' health histories, it is important to interpret the information provided by careful questioning.

- The aim of treatment is to understand how patients are functioning in their environment and how their dental needs and treatment fit into their lifestyle.

- Rational treatment planning philosophy can guide the development of treatment alternatives, by using evidence-based data, where available, and selecting alternatives that are compatible with a patient's lifestyle and general health-modifying factors.

- Some of the alternatives to the treatment of caries for frail and functionally dependent older adults, especially those with severe cognitive impairment, are incomplete caries removal followed by sealing the lesions with glass ionomer. SDF also can be used to arrest caries in this population.

DISCLOSURE

The authors have nothing to disclose.

REFERENCES

1. Roberts AW, Ogunwole SU, Blackslee L, et al. The population over 65 years and older in the United States:2016. Washington, DC: Bureau UC; 2016.

2. Nelson EA, Dannefer D. Aged heterogeneity: fact or fiction? The fate of diversity in gerontological research. Gerontologist 1992;32(1):17–23.
3. Ettinger RL, Beck JD. The new elderly: what can the dental profession expect? Spec Care Dentist 1982;2(2):62–9.
4. Marchini L, Hartshorn JE, Cowen H, et al. A teaching tool for establishing risk of oral health deterioration in elderly patients: development, implementation, and evaluation at a U.S. dental school. J Dent Educ 2017;81(11):1283–90.
5. Ettinger RL. Treatment planning concepts for the ageing patient. Aust Dent J 2015;60(Suppl 1):71–85.
6. Marchini L, Reynolds JC, Caplan DJ, et al. Predictors of having a dentist among older adults in Iowa. Community Dent Oral Epidemiol 2020;48(3):240–7.
7. Flick K, Marchini L. The interprofessional role in dental caries management: from the social worker perspective. Dent Clin North Am 2019;63(4):663–8.
8. Montini T, Tseng TY, Patel H, et al. Barriers to dental services for older adults. Am J Health Behav 2014;38(5):781–8.
9. Mulligan R, Vanderlinde MA. Treating the older adult dental patient: what are the issues of concern? J Calif Dent Assoc 2009;37(11):804–10.
10. Marchini L, Ettinger RL. COVID-19 pandemics and oral health care for older adults. Spec Care Dentist 2020;40(3):329–31.
11. Chávez EM, Ship JA. Sensory and motor deficits in the elderly: impact on oral health. J Public Health Dent 2000;60(4):297–303.
12. Kurlander J, Saini S. Virtual visits: telehealth and older adults. National Poll on Healthy Aging. Ann Arbor: University of Michigan; 2019.
13. Tynan A, Deeth L, McKenzie D, et al. Integrated approach to oral health in aged care facilities using oral health practitioners and teledentistry in rural Queensland. Aust J Rural Health 2018;26:290–4.
14. León S, Giacaman RA. COVID-19 and inequities in oral health care for older people: an opportunity for emerging paradigms. JDR Clin Trans Res 2020;5(4): 290–2.
15. McGee J. Things to know if your written material is for older adults. In: McGee J, editor. Toolkit for making written material clear and effective. 1st edition. Washington, DC: Centers for Medicare & Medicaid Services; 2010. p. 1–10.
16. Peres MA, Macpherson LMD, Weyant RJ, et al. Oral diseases: a global public health challenge. Lancet 2019;394(10194):249–60.
17. Murray Thomson W. Epidemiology of oral health conditions in older people. Gerodontology 2014;31(Suppl 1):9–16.
18. Lopez R, Smith PC, Gostemeyer G, et al. Ageing, dental caries and periodontal diseases. J Clin Periodontol 2017;44(Suppl 18):S145–52.
19. Berkey DB. Clinical decision-making for the geriatric dental patient. Gerodontics 1988;4(6):321–6.
20. Ettinger RL. Rational dental care: part 1. Has the concept changed in 20 years? J Can Dent Assoc 2006;72(5):441–5.
21. Ettinger R, Beck JD, Jakobsen J. The development of teaching programs in geriatric dentistry in the United States from 1974 to 1979. Spec Care Dentist 1981; 1(5):221–4.
22. Doyle DJ, Goyal A, Bansal P, et al. American Society of Anesthesiologists Classification (ASA class). In: Doyle DJ, Goyal A, Bansal P, et al, editors. StatPearls. Treasure Island (FL): StatPearls Publishing LLC; 2020. StatPearls Publishing Copyright © 2020.
23. Kamen S. The resolution of oral health care for the institutionalized geriatric patient. Spec Care Dentist 1983;3(6):249–50.

24. Gordon SR, Kress GC Jr. Treatment planning in dental schools. J Dent Educ 1987;51(5):224–8.
25. Laudenbach JM. Treatment planning for the geriatric patient. In: Laudenbach JMS, Ship JA, editors. Clinicians guide to oral health in geriatric patients. 3rd edition. Washington, DC: Amer Acad Of Oral Medicine; 2010. p. 7–8.
26. Shay K. Identifying the needs of the elderly dental patient. The geriatric dental assessment. Dent Clin North Am 1994;38(3):499–523.
27. Berkey DB, Berg RG, Ettinger RL, et al. The old-old dental patient: the challenge of clinical decision-making. J Am Dent Assoc 1996;127(3):321–32.
28. Johnson TE, Shuman SK, Ofstehage JC. Fitting the pieces together: treatment planning in the geriatric dental patient. Dent Clin North Am 1997;41(4):945–59.
29. Dye BA, Weatherspoon DJ, Lopez Mitnik G. Tooth loss among older adults according to poverty status in the United States from 1999 through 2004 and 2009 through 2014. J Am Dent Assoc 2019;150(1):9–23.e3.
30. Featherstone JD, Doméjean S. Minimal intervention dentistry: part 1. From 'compulsive' restorative dentistry to rational therapeutic strategies. Br Dent J 2012;213(9):441–5.
31. Chalmers JM. Minimal intervention dentistry: part 1. Strategies for addressing the new caries challenge in older patients. J Can Dent Assoc 2006;72(5):427–33.
32. Li R, Lo EC, Liu BY, et al. Randomized clinical trial on arresting dental root caries through silver diammine fluoride applications in community-dwelling elders. J Dent 2016;51:15–20.
33. da Mata C, Allen PF, McKenna G, et al. Two-year survival of ART restorations placed in elderly patients: a randomised controlled clinical trial. J Dent 2015; 43(4):405–11.
34. da Mata C, Allen PF, Cronin M, et al. Cost-effectiveness of ART restorations in elderly adults: a randomized clinical trial. Community Dent Oral Epidemiol 2014;42(1):79–87.
35. Gluzman R, Katz RV, Frey BJ, et al. Prevention of root caries: a literature review of primary and secondary preventive agents. Spec Care Dentist 2013;33(3):133–40.
36. Käyser AF. Shortened dental arches and oral function. J Oral Rehabil 1981;8(5): 457–62.
37. Kern JS, Wolfart S, Hilgers RD, et al. The randomized shortened dental arch study: influence of two different treatments on interdental spacing over 5 years. Clin Oral Investig 2017;21(6):1945–51.
38. McKenna G, Allen F, Woods N, et al. Cost-effectiveness of tooth replacement strategies for partially dentate elderly: a randomized controlled clinical trial. Community Dent Oral Epidemiol 2014;42(4):366–74.
39. Fueki K, Baba K. Shortened dental arch and prosthetic effect on oral health-related quality of life: a systematic review and meta-analysis. J Oral Rehabil 2017;44(7):563–72.
40. Jayaratne YS, Zwahlen RA. The evolution of dental journals from 2003 to 2012: a bibliometric analysis. PLoS One 2015;10(3):e0119503.
41. De Visschere LM, van der Putten GJ, Vanobbergen JN, et al, Dutch Association of Nursing Home Physicians. An oral health care guideline for institutionalised older people. Gerodontology 2011;28(4):307–10.
42. Marchini L, Ettinger R, Hartshorn J. Personalized dental caries management for frail older adults and persons with special needs. Dent Clin North Am 2019; 63(4):631–51.
43. Chalmers J, Pearson A. Oral hygiene care for residents with dementia: a literature review. J Adv Nurs 2005;52(4):410–9.

Interdisciplinary Education and Health Care in Geriatric Dental Medicine

Matthew Mara, DMD, EdM

KEYWORDS

- Geriatric dental medicine • Interprofessional education (IPE) • Collaborative practice
- Team-based care

KEY POINTS

- With the increasing number of older patients with natural dentition and complex medical needs, communicating and collaborating with other health care providers will be paramount in providing comprehensive dental care in the twenty-first century.
- There is a growing need for health professional programs to provide students with interprofessional education (IPE) experiences to prepare their graduates for the workforce.
- Geriatrics provides an excellent channel for IPE experiences, resulting in improved patient outcomes of some of the most vulnerable members of society.
- Existing models of interprofessional practice in geriatrics such as adult day programs, nursing homes, long-term care facilities, home care, and simulated learning experiences are avenues to implement IPE experiences.
- Continuing education (CE) programs across the health professions should consider offering training and CE credit for learning skills in IPE and collaborative practice for all members of the dental community.

INTRODUCTION

Have you noticed a shift in the age of your patients? Or, are you making fewer dentures than you thought you would in your practice? Whether you acknowledge it or not, your patient population is likely aging, primarily if you practice outside of a densely populated urban area. As the US population ages, so do their dentition; however, the clinical presentation of elderly dentition looks different than it did even half a century ago. Rates of edentulism are declining, and an increasing number of patients are maintaining their natural dentition well into their golden years.[1] A general dentist will likely encounter a geriatric patient weekly, if not daily, in their practice. Elderly patients are more likely

This article originally appeared in Dental Clinics, Volume 65 Issue 2, April 2021.
Department of General Dentistry, Boston University Henry M. Goldman School of Dental Medicine, 560 Harrison Avenue, Room 325, Boston, MA, USA
E-mail address: maramb@bu.edu

Clin Geriatr Med 39 (2023) 327–341
https://doi.org/10.1016/j.cger.2023.01.006
geriatric.theclinics.com

to have complex medical needs that may require a different approach to care. As dentistry becomes more accustomed to treating medically compromised geriatric patients, providing comprehensive, collaborative care will become standard practice.

Collaboration among health care professionals has demonstrated benefits of improved patient outcomes.[2] Despite knowledge of patient benefits, often, in practice, health care specialties operate in silos with minimal communication and coordination of patient care.[3] Although the benefits of collaborative care are known for patients throughout their lifetime, geriatric patients may benefit from the partnership between health care providers due to their significant medical needs.[4] To address this gap, professional organizations such as the American Medical Association have called for increased collaboration between members of the health care team.[5] As a response, health professional education programs across the disciplines have started to implement interprofessional education (IPE) requirements to model collaborative patient care experiences for students. These experiences aim to graduate a new generation of health care professionals equipped with valuable collaborative knowledge and skills to enter the workforce and become meaningful contributors to the patient care team.

As this chapter explores the role of IPE in geriatric dental medicine, the hope is that you will acknowledge the limitations of a 'uni-professional identity,' one which isolates the dental profession and by nature and generates misunderstandings amongst healthcare providers and establish a 'multi-professional identity'.[6] Failure to develop a dentist's view as a partner in collaborative person-centered practice can propagate negative stereotypes between health care professionals and ultimately negatively affect patient care.[6] By viewing the role of a dentist more broadly, as a valued contributor to a patient's health care team, the hope is to improve patient outcomes and prepare the dental profession for the health care delivery system of the future.

INTERPROFESSIONAL EDUCATION

IPE is a purposeful, planned interaction between health professional students of different disciplines. The World Health Organization and the Center for the Advancement of Interprofessional Education define IPE as the learning experience that "occurs when two or more professions (students, residents and health workers) learn with, about, and from each other to enable effective collaboration and improve health outcomes."[7] A Health Resources and Services Administration report indicated that interdisciplinary education best exists in collaborative teams where (1) teams work to address a sizable complex problem where no one individual can create a solution alone, (2) teams represent a variety of fields that will make solving the problem easier, (3) all contributors' skills and knowledge are considered equally as important, and (4) team members share a collective goal.[8]

Early attempts to provide interprofessional experiences for health professional students included educating students from different health professions together through combined courses and voluntary educational experiences.[9] Elective or happenstance types of IPE experiences are not as effective as carefully crafted experiences designed to provide collaborative training. Cahn (2014) argues how interprofessional skills must be strategic and well planned to maximize their effect.[9] These findings suggest that IPE experiences require a carefully selected, specific, and permanent place in the health profession curriculum. Accrediting bodies of dental, medical, and nursing programs, among many others, include accreditation standards requiring institutions to provide IPE experiences. **Table 1** outlines the IPE accreditation requirements of the Commission on Dental Accreditation (CODA), Liaison Committee on Medical Education (LCME), and the Commission on Colligate Nursing Education (CCNE). Similar

Table 1 Interprofessional education accreditation standards in dentistry, medicine, and nursing	
	Accreditation Standards
Dentistry	"2–20 Graduates must be competent in communicating and collaborating with other members of the health care team to facilitate the provision of health care. Intent: In attaining competence, students should understand the roles of members of the health care team and have educational experiences, particularly clinical experiences that involve working with other healthcare professional students and practitioners. Students should have educational experiences in which they coordinate patient care within the health care system relevant to dentistry."[10]
Medicine	"7.9 Interprofessional Collaborative Skills The faculty of a medical school ensure that the core curriculum of the medical education program prepares medical students to function collaboratively on health care teams that include health professionals from other disciplines as they provide coordinated services to patients. These curricular experiences include practitioners and/or students from other health professions."[11]
Nursing	"III-H The curriculum includes planned clinical practice experiences that: a) enable students to integrate new knowledge and demonstrate attainment of program outcomes, b) foster interprofessional collaborative practice and c) are evaluated by faculty."[12]

standards have emerged in pharmacy, physical therapy, physician assistant, dietician, and social work programs to ensure administration craft collaborative opportunities within their curriculum.

Because IPE earns a permanent spot in the health profession curricula, professional schools will produce new graduates more experienced and prepared for collaborative practice. Although team-based collaborative care is not a new concept for nursing and medical programs, dental programs have started to include IPE experiences within the last decade in response to changes in CODA accreditation standards.[13] Often, IPE experiences are part of special care or pediatric courses and clinics. Demonstrated benefits of increasing student knowledge, confidence, and clinical practice have been shown in pediatric IPE experiences.[14] In addition, significant changes in students' attitudes toward IPE and collaborative care are known results of geriatric training programs.[15] Regardless of which courses dental schools use to incorporate IPE into their curriculum, collaborative practice should start early and occur often in dental students' training.[15] Dental schools may consider IPE programs to partner with other health professional programs to reduce disparities in the frail and community-dwelling elderly.

Interprofessional Education and the Geriatric Patient

Older adults may benefit significantly from an interdisciplinary team-based approach to care, as geriatric patients are more likely to have multiple medical comorbidities and physical and cognitive impairments.[16] Managing various health concerns adds additional layers of complexity for providers of geriatric patients, as risks and benefits of treatment options need careful evaluation in the treatment planning process. Models of collaborative care in geriatrics are known to aid health care teams in prioritizing patient-specific care plans. Initial multidisciplinary team assessments have shown improved patient outcome measures for geriatric patients over time.[17] Therefore, the geriatrics curriculum is ideal for professional schools to integrate IPE and significantly affect patient quality of life and health outcomes.

Models of IPE experiences readily exist in geriatric education and training across the disciplines. Authentic IPE experiences expand beyond providing care within a multidisciplinary network and allow students to collaborate on interdisciplinary teams to address complex patient problems.[18] Medical geriatric training programs have a strong history of promoting interdisciplinary and collaborative care, whereas evidence is more variable in other health professional programs.[19] Dentists should communicate with geriatricians and learn from their approach to collaborative practice. Dental schools should consider including IPE experiences in geriatrics throughout the dental curricula to best prepare students for future practice.[19]

Successful Interdisciplinary Care Requires Teamwork

As a practicing dentist, you are no stranger to the importance and value of teamwork. Similar to how your dental team's success relies on all members having clearly defined roles, understanding others' roles, and working together to achieve a shared mission, interdisciplinary care and IPE experiences also rely on teamwork.[20] A key component of successful collaborative care is that groups understand the roles and responsibilities of all collaborators as they establish and work toward a common goal.[21] Therefore, interdisciplinary groups should set agreed-on rules and create standards of communication, with plans that will allow members to identify and resolve conflict when it arises.[22] It is considered best practice to spend some time acquainting one another with specific roles and establishing protocols and guidelines once interdisciplinary teams form.

In addition, similar to how a general dentist relies on all team members' flexibility, members of interprofessional care teams need to demonstrate flexibility with changing circumstances. It is considered good practice for interdisciplinary teams to establish a means to receive feedback and provide performance reviews to improve the team's function. Feedback can be a successful way to identify successes and isolate growth opportunities, making the team-based approach to care more efficacious.

Lastly, the collaborative approach should consider patients' desires through shared decision-making. Finding common ground can be challenging when team members have different beliefs of what shared decision-making is or what shared decision looks like in their specialty.[23] Although the concept of shared decision-making is evolving in geriatrics, collaborative teams should work to identify patient's values and goals, as they collectively construct a plan of care.[24] In geriatric dental medicine, there are endless examples of shared decision-making related to providing treatment or not providing treatment to our most vulnerable and frail elders. In practice, this may translate to a conversation with a patient's family and interprofessional team to decide to collectively monitor and apply periodic fluoride to a calcified root tip in a 92-year-old patient, instead of extraction. It may also mean relining an old set of worn dentures with porcelain teeth instead of making them new dentures based on the patient's esthetic preference and likeliness to comply with treatment. Regardless of the level of shared decision-making, all members of the patient's care team must be on board with the decision to provide or monitor specific treatment options, especially when the decision has the potential to affect the care of multiple members of the team.

Teamwork is essential for effective interdisciplinary care. It is crucial if you are interested in forming or joining a collaborative care team to set aside time to create common goals, be open and receptive to feedback, communicate effectively, and participate in shared decision-making with patients, patient families, and caretakers.

Establishing Excellent Collaborative Care Models Is Challenging

Regardless of the inherent benefits of collaborative care in geriatrics, institutions and programs face many challenges when designing interdisciplinary experiences.[19] Known problems associated with the design and implementation of IPE in health professional programs are seen in **Fig. 1**.[9,18,25] The challenges listed in **Fig. 1** apply to providing students with IPE experience in health professional programs but also applying collaborative care in clinical practice.

Two specific challenges are associated with implementing IPE experiences to highlight (1) the lack of experienced dental faculty[18] and (2) status differences among different health care disciplines.[18] These challenges make it more difficult for dental schools to establish active IPE experiences for their students and create potential roadblocks to collaborative care in their future practice.

Although IPE in dentistry is considered an emerging practice, dentists who have significant exposure to meaningful collaboration with professionals across disciplines are uniquely poised to become leaders in IPE in academia. These practitioners may seek partnerships with dental schools or dental organizations to provide IPE experiences to students or offer examples of effective collaborative care to practicing dentists.

Status differences in health care disciplines can present a challenge for designing IPE experiences in health professional programs and establishing effective collaborative

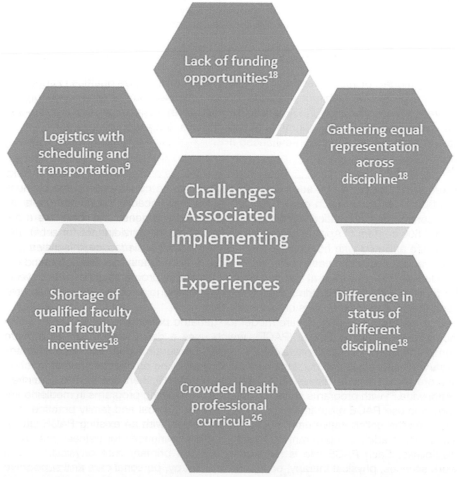

Fig. 1. Challenges associated with the implementation of interprofessional learning experiences.

care teams in practice. The American Dental Association Action for Dental Health Initiative offers strategies that dentists can use to collaborate with other health professionals and bridge disciplines. Suggestions from the Health Resources and Service Administration include (1) developing relationships with local physicians and pediatricians for referrals, (2) taking body mass index of the patient and referring patients to primary care if they are at risk of being overweight, and (3) collaboration with pediatricians to apply fluoride varnish and/or refer children with high caries risk.[26] Although these strategies may not eliminate the potential for status-related challenges in interprofessional teams, it opens up communication lines. In addition, it demonstrates to other health care providers the potential for meaningful collaboration with dental professionals.

Gaining additional insight from practicing dentists who participate in interdisciplinary patient care is essential for the widespread, long-term effects of IPE. Even though professional programs in dentistry, medicine, nursing, social work, pharmacy, and psychology have IPE experiences within their curriculum, many consider existing IPE experiences inadequate to graduate a workforce ready to make interdisciplinary team care a priority.[27] Therefore, health professional programs must form meaningful partnerships with community stakeholders to offer optimal IPE experiences.[25] Existing interdisciplinary practice models in geriatrics may provide an avenue for dental schools and practicing dentists to develop relevant collaborative care skills.

EXISTING MODELS OF INTERDISCIPLINARY PRACTICE FOR GERIATRIC PATIENTS

Existing models of interprofessional education and collaborative practice in geriatrics are readily available within health professional education programs and health care delivery systems across North America. This section explores examples of collaborative practice in adult day programs, nursing homes, long-term care facilities, home care programs, and simulation-enhanced IPE.

Day Programs

There were close to 4,600 adult day centers across the country that serve close to 300,000 older adults each day in 2010.[28] In the last decade, the number of adult day centers has dramatically increased; reports now suggest that there are more than 7,500 centers.[29] Approximately 70% of adult day centers are not-for-profit and most are affiliated with home care, medical centers, or skilled nursing facilities and offer various social and health services.[30] Projections suggest that 74% of attendees of adult day programs live at home,[31] which makes day programs accessible options for families who serve as primary caretakers, as these programs are known to help ease the burden of caregivers on older adults.[32]

One existing collaborative care model for geriatric patients is the Program of All-inclusive Care for the Elderly (PACE), which uses a day center model to provide comprehensive and collaborative care. The PACE program's goal is to reduce unnecessary hospital stays and nursing home care by focusing on maintenance of function and prevention of acute disease.[33] As of September 2019, there are 263 PACE centers nationwide,[34] with programs spanning 36 states.[35] Training programs in medicine are known to use PACE programs as rotation sites for medical and family practice residents on the collaborative care model.[36] Partnership with an existing PACE site or similar elder adult day program could afford IPE experiences for trainees across all disciplines. Each PACE site is required to have a primary care physician, social work services, physical therapy, occupational therapy, personal care and supportive therapies, nutritional counseling, recreational theory, and meals.[37] Although geriatric dentists are not essential members of the collaborative team, PACE programs readily offer dental services and include dentists in patient care conferences.[38] Often this includes partnering with a community dentist. Occasionally, this includes providing dental services on-site, affording more significant interaction between dental professionals and other members of the patient care team. Physically including dentistry within PACE programs sites could allow community dentists to shadow, network, and refer complex medically compromised geriatric patients. Dental schools may also seek partnerships with local PACE programs to expose students to a model of collaborative team-based care in geriatrics.

Nursing Homes

Nursing homes and facilities for community-dwelling elders present another avenue for collaborative geriatric patient care.[39] Interdisciplinary care is essential in nursing facilities, as the increased collaborative practices in these environments have shown increased health outcomes.[40] The percentage of older adults living in nursing homes decreased over the last two decades, as the priority focuses on keeping elders residing within the community. Today approximately 4.5% of adults older than 65 years live in nursing homes,[41] which suggests that older adults living in nursing home facilities have complex needs and would benefit from a team-based approach to care.

Examples of IPE in nursing home facilities exist within the United States; however, they are not distributed evenly in all areas or across all populations. There is a lack of geriatric IPE experiences in settings of community-dwelling older adults in underserved areas.[19] This gap in services presents an opportunity for health professional institutions to partner with nursing homes to establish educational training centers that could foster collaboration between dental, medical, nursing, pharmacy and social work students. These programs would allow students to work together to treat some of our nation's most vulnerable older adults.[39] Dental and dental hygiene students may play an essential role in nursing facilities.

Studies suggest that the burden of oral health disease in the population of community-dwelling older adults is high, and a significant need for oral health promotion programs exists.[42] Practicing dentists may seek opportunities to volunteer or provide meaningful services in nursing homes in their community by providing dental services and/or oral health education to older adults, their families, and nursing home staff.

Long-Term Care Facilities

Older individuals in long-term care facilities typically suffer from chronic conditions, trauma, or illnesses that interfere with their ability to complete activities of daily living (ALDs).[43] ALDs include household chores, preparing meals, managing finances, and personal hygiene, such as proper tooth brushing or caring for dentures. Health care goals in long-term care facilities no longer focus on curing an individual's illnesses. Instead, they focus on maintaining a maximum level of function. While developing patient care plans in long term care facilities, it is essential that care teams consider an individual's oral health condition, especially as it relates to their ability and willingness to chew and eat food. This plays a significant role in a geriatric patient's care plan, as individuals with chronic illness are more likely to be undernourished and lack vital nutrients in their diet.[44] Offering dental students training in this collaborative setting is critical, as they weigh the risks and benefits of an ideal dental treatment plan. This environment may also emphasize shared decision-making and collaborative care with the patients' health care team and family. Developing modified treatment plans is an essential skill that health profession students could practice through collaborative experiences in long-term care facilities. Because these patients have significantly complex medical teams, long-term care facilities often have extensive provider networks, making them an excellent resource for training new professional students and providing practicing professionals exposure to collaborative care models.

Home Care

Home care is an additional avenue to provide trainees with experience in collaborative, interdisciplinary care. By 2050 more than 27 million people in the United States will be living at home and need some help with ADLs.[44] For that reason, a substantial increase in home health care jobs will be available to meet this growing need, and the US Health professional training programs should develop training experiences in treating patients outside of a typical clinical setting.[45] Home care interdisciplinary team visits have demonstrated benefits for medical, physician assistant, occupational theory, social work, physical therapy, pharmacy, and dental students.[15] Continuing education training experiences in home-based care for dental professionals may be a way to expand at home services for older patients and expose practitioners to best practices and professional standards when treating patients outside of the typical dental setting.

Simulation-Enhanced Interprofessional Education

One model that allows students and clinicians to gain experience and practice in inter-disciplinary collaborative outside of the patient care experience is through simulation-enhanced learning activities. The goal of simulation-enhanced IPE experiences is to provide opportunities for training and learning in collaborative care while offering trainees opportunities for evaluation and reflection.[46] Simulation-enhanced IPE makes use of a simulator such as a standardized patient, mannequin, avatar, or virtual, proce-dural, or computer-based model,[46] minimizing many of the physical barriers that exist when designing collaborative patient-based experiences. Simulation-enhanced IPE may be a way for health professional programs to provide valuable IPE experiences to students in a remote learning environment. Benefits of simulation-enhanced IPE include (1) similarities to clinical practice, (2) objective scoring opportunities through a comprehensive evaluation of team and individual performance, (3) opportunity to provide meaningful feedback, and (4) reflection and ability to design a variety of simulations to meet specific program's needs.[47]

Health professional education programs are unique in their ability to incorporate simulation-enhanced IPE experiences into their curriculum and continuing education programs through their simulation learning centers. These simulated learning environments may provide schools with space and resources when designing interprofessional experiences with other health professional programs. Simulated learning environments of dental schools or other health professional programs may serve as ideal locations for interprofessional training for practicing clinicians who seek learning opportunities for the best practices of collaborative care. Conducting virtual IPE training experiences may also expose clinicians to best practices when training centers are not available within their community.

Table 2 summarizes pertinent characteristics, services available, and opportunities for collaborating care for day programs, nursing homes, long-term care facilities, home visits, and simulation-enhanced IPE experiences.

Day programs, nursing homes, long-term care facilities, home care, and virtual simulation are models of interprofessional practice for geriatric patients. The role the dentist plays in these collaborative environments varies by program and available resources. In partnership with dental schools and American Dental Education Association, the dental profession needs to continue to develop and endorse collaborative models of overall care for this vulnerable population and highlight successful programs to serve as models and best practices for other institutions.

Table 2
Existing models of geriatric interdisciplinary care and suggestions for expanding collaborative practice

	Day Programs	Nursing Homes	Long-Term Care Facilities	Home Visits	Simulation-Enhanced IPE
Pertinent characteristics of care	They are designed mostly for older adults living at home. The goal is to minimize hospital stays and move to nursing home or long-term care facilities. Modifications from the ideal dental treatment plan may not be needed.	Community-dwelling elders with complex medical needs that benefit from team-based care. The number of older adults living in nursing homes is decreasing nationally. Modifications from an ideal treatment plan may or may not be needed.	Community members need assistance with ADLs. Less focus on curing illness, a greater emphasis on maintaining function. Because of complex medical needs, most treatment plans will require deviations from the ideal.	Homebound patients, typically receiving care from family or home health care aids. Should be reserved for patients who have difficulty or are unable to leave their home. Modifications from an ideal treatment plan are likely due to limitations of providing care inside a patient's home.	Can be done anywhere and at any time. Uses standardized patients that can have varying levels of medical needs. Relies on education technology.
Available health care services	Primary care, nursing, nursing aids, physical therapists, occupational therapists, social work, transportation services, nutrition counseling, recreational therapy, emergency services, pharmacy, dentistry.	Primary care, nursing, nursing aids, physical therapists, occupational therapists, nutritional support, pharmacy social work, dentistry.	Primary care, nursing, nursing aids, volunteer care, nutritional support, physical therapists, occupational therapists, pharmacy, social work, dentistry.	Nursing, nursing aids, personal care aides, physical therapists, occupational therapists, speech and language pathologists, social work services, nutritional support, companionship, volunteer care, transportation services, pharmacy, dentistry.	Multiple medical disciplines, nursing, allied health, pharmacy, dentistry, are limitless as new simulation experiences emerge.

(continued on next page)

Table 2
(continued)

	Day Programs	Nursing Homes	Long-Term Care Facilities	Home Visits	Simulation-Enhanced IPE
Opportunities for collaborative care	Form partnerships between dental schools, community dentists, and PACE sites/other nonprofit day centers.	Expand existing training programs to more readily include dentistry. Seek partnerships with local nursing facilities to provide education to patients, families, and staff.	Partner with existing networks and training centers. Include dental providers in patient care conferences and provide opportunities for shared decision-making with other providers and caretakers.	Need for dental professional organizations to sponsor CE on regulations and best practices for practicing dentists interested in home visits and at-home care.	Expand technology and resources within dental schools to increase simulation-based learning with other health professional students. Encourage continuing education offerings for practicing dentists in simulation-enhanced IPE.

INTERPROFESSIONAL EDUCATION MODELS IN HEALTH PROFESSION EDUCATION

There is a clear need for effective models of interprofessional practice in geriatrics, even within existing health care delivery systems. The Interprofessional Education Collaborative (IPEC) was established in 2009 between the professional education organizations of six health professional fields (allopathic medicine, osteopathic medicine, dentistry, nursing, pharmacy, and public health) to guide curriculum and development in collaborative care in the health professions. IPEC has established four competency domains designed to be present from professional training and expand throughout clinical practice. IPEC competency domains include (1) teamwork and team-based practices, (2) communication practices, (3) values and ethics, and (4) roles and responsibilities.[48] Organizations such as the National Center for Interprofessional Practice and Education and the American Interprofessional Health Collaborative provide resources on programs that promote interprofessional education and practice that use IPEC competencies. This article explores the Program for Interprofessional Practice and Education (PIPE) at the University of California San Francisco[49] and the Michigan Center for Interprofessional Education[50] to provide examples on how dental schools are adjusting their curricula to incorporate meaningful IPE experiences across all years of their programs.

The Program for Interprofessional Practice and Education at University of California San Francisco

The PIPE program at the University of California San Francisco provides a collaborative learning space for dental, medical, pharmacy, nursing, and physical therapy students. The PIPE program's interprofessional collaborative care framework uses IPEC competencies. It outlines experiences where students are exposed to, immersed in, and become more competent in IPE, moving toward proficiency in clinical practice. The PIPE program conducts an initial baseline assessment on student skills before their first exposure. It then provides formative assessment opportunities in immersive experiences throughout the curricula and concludes with summative assessments on IPE competencies. When outlining IPE experiences in other health professional schools and programs, institutions should develop similar curriculum maps. This structure ensures that schools introduce, practice, and assess collaborative skills across the students' academic experiences to best prepare them for their future practice.

Michigan Center for Interprofessional Education

The Michigan Center for Interprofessional Education provides IPE experiences for students across multiple professional programs with the motto "Better together."[50] They offer a variety of IPE courses for students, in addition to interprofessional leadership workshops for all health professional faculty and a fellowship program for faculty leaders who propose and complete collaborative research and training projects. One example of the courses supported by the center is Geriatric Medicine—a team-based approach for medical and pharmacy students, which provides students with practice on all four IPEC competencies.[50] Dental schools and professional organizations may consider establishing centers for IPE and designing programs for both students and faculty on best practices.

MOVING FORWARD: A SHIFT TO INTERPROFESSIONAL GERIATRIC PRACTICE

Dental professionals need to shift from a solo-based medical practice model to a multidisciplinary and team-based approach. Although IPE experiences are becoming more ubiquitous in dental education, practicing dentists may desire and benefit from opportunities to engage with other health care professionals. The shift toward interprofessional practice may help dental organizations and agencies provide continuing education credits outlining best practices and models for team-based care. Providing continuing education credits may be of increased importance, as the dental profession explores value-based reimbursement. Although widespread value-based reimbursement in dentistry is far in the distance, pilot programs in group practices and community health centers will be implemented where collaborative interdisciplinary care may increase efficiency and lower overall costs.[51]

As dental organizations grow to better understand the dentist's role in interprofessional practice, it may be possible that these organizations could develop training modules to improve the overall care of the vulnerable geriatric population. Professionally recognized training modules or programs can then be replicated and used by dental schools and dental organizations to prepare dental professionals to best make a meaningful impact through interprofessional practice.

SUMMARY

As of 2019, fewer than 40% of practicing dentists in the United States are younger than 44 years.[52] This means that it is likely that more than 60% of practicing US dentists professional training did not include training in IPE. Although the benefits of IPE and collaborative practice are known to improve patient outcomes, most practicing dentists need professional development opportunities to formally develop skills and learn best practices. As IPE becomes a more prominent component of health professional education and health care delivery systems, practicing dentists should seek opportunities to collaborate with other health professional colleagues to best treat shared patients. With the growing aging population in the United States and the complex medical considerations that go along with providing geriatric care, practicing dentists should consider ways to collaborate with other health professionals as an essential way to best treat this vulnerable population.

CLINICS CARE POINTS

- Do not hesitate to communicate with other health care professionals when planning and rendering treatment to older patients.
- Involve your patient and their health care proxy when considering treatment options and expected outcomes.
- Seek opportunities to refine and further develop collaborative skills and team-based training.
- Introduce yourself and your practice to area health care providers to foster interdisciplinary networks to referrals and consultations.
- Volunteer your time in local nursing homes and long-term care facilities providing oral health education to patients, families, and staff to facilitate a team-based approach.

DISCLOSURES

The author declares no conflict of interest. Personal views are that of the author and not that of Boston University.

REFERENCES

1. Douglass CW, Shih A, Ostry L. Will there be a need for complete dentures in the United States in 2020? J Prosthet Dent 2002;87(1):5–8.
2. Martin J, Ummenhofer W, Manser T, et al. Interprofessional collaboration among nurses and physicians: Making a difference in patient outcome. Swiss Med Wkly 2010;140:w13062.
3. Margalit R, Thompson S, Visovsky C, et al. From professional silos to interprofessional education. Qual Manag Health Care 2009;18(3):165–73.
4. Moore A, Patterson C, White J, et al. Interprofessional and integrated care of the elderly in a family health team. 2020. Available at: https://www.cfp.ca/content/58/8/e436.short. Accessed July 2, 2020.
5. American Medical Association. Making the case for interprofessional education. 2020. Available at: https://www.ama-assn.org/education/accelerating-change-medical-education/making-case-interprofessional-education. Accessed July 14, 2020.
6. Khalili H, Hall J, DeLuca S. Historical analysis of professionalism in western societies: implications for interprofessional education and collaborative practice. J Interprof Care 2014;28(2):92–7.
7. National center for interprofessional practice and education. About IPE. 2020. Available at: https://nexusipe.org/informing/about-ipe. Accessed July 14, 2020.
8. Klein J. 48202 Library Trends. Interdisciplinary studies program, vol. 45. Detroit (MI): Wayne State University; 1996. p. 13454. No. 2, Fall.
9. Cahn PS. In and out of the curriculum: an historical case study in implementing interprofessional education. J Interprof Care 2014;28(2):128–33.
10. Commission on dental accreditation. Accreditation standards for dental education programs, p. 28. 2016. Available at: http://www.ada.org/~/media/CODA/Files/predoc.ashx. Accessed July 14, 2020.
11. Liaison committee on medical education. Functions and structure of medical school, p. 11. Available at: https://lcme.org/publications/. Accessed July 14, 2020.
12. Commission on colligate education. (2018) Accreditation standards of bachlarriate and graduate nursing programs, p. 16. Available at: https://www.aacnnursing.org/Portals/42/CCNE/PDF/Standards-Final-2018.pdf. Accessed July 20, 2020.
13. Hamil LM. Looking back to move ahead: interprofessional education in dental education. J Dent Educ 2017;81(8):eS74–80.
14. Cooper D, Kim J, Duderstadt K, et al. Interprofessional oral health education improves knowledge, confidence, and practice for pediatric healthcare providers. Front Public Health 2017;5. https://doi.org/10.3389/fpubh.2017.00209.
15. Reilly JM, Aranda MP, Segal-Gidan F, et al. Assessment of student interprofessional education (IPE) training for team-based geriatric home care: does IPE training change students' knowledge and attitudes? Home Health Care Serv Q 2014;33(4):177–93.
16. American Geriatrics Society. Patient-centered care for older adults with multiple chronic conditions: a stepwise approach. J Am Geriatr Soc 2012;60(10):1957–68.
17. Burns R, Nichols LO, Martindale-Adams J, et al. Interdisciplinary geriatric primary care evaluation and management: two-year outcomes. J Am Geriatr Soc 2000;48(1):8–13.
18. Skinner JH. Transitioning from multidisciplinary to interdisciplinary education in gerontology and geriatrics. Gerontol Geriatr Educ 2001;21(3):73–85.

19. Schapmire TJ, Head BA, Nash WA, et al. Overcoming barriers to interprofessional education in gerontology: the interprofessional curriculum for the care of older adults. Adv Med Educ Pract 2018;9:109–18.

20. Kagan SH. Revisiting interdisciplinary teamwork in geriatric acute care. Geriatr Nurs 2010;31(2):133–6.

21. Youngwerth J, Twaddle M. Cultures of interdisciplinary teams: how to foster good dynamics. J Palliat Med 2011;14(5):650–4.

22. Drinka T. Interdisciplinary geriatric teams: approaches to conflict as indicators of potential to model teamwork. Educ Gerontol 1994;20(1):87–103.

23. Chong WW, Aslani P, Chen TF. Multiple perspectives on shared decision-making and interprofessional collaboration in mental healthcare. J Interprof Care 2013; 27(3):223–30.

24. Van de Pol MHJ, Fluit CRMG, Lagro J, et al. Expert and patient consensus on a dynamic model for shared decision-making in frail older patients. Patient Educ Couns 2016;99(6):1069–77.

25. Reuben DB, Yee MN, Cole KD, et al. Organizational issues in establishing geriatrics interdisciplinary team training. Gerontol Geriatr Educ 2004;24(2):13–34.

26. Health Resources and Services Administration. Considerations for oral health integration in primary care practice for children. Available at: https://www.hrsa.gov/sites/default/files/oralhealth/oralhealthprimarychildren.pdf. Accessed July 14, 2020.

27. Partnership for Health in Aging Workgroup on Interdisciplinary Team Training in Geriatrics. Position statement on interdisciplinary team training in geriatrics: an essential component of quality health care for older adults. J Am Geriatr Soc 2014;62(5):961–5.

28. National Adult Day Services Administration. Research. Available at: https://www.nadsa.org/research/#:%7E:text=Adult%20day%20centers%20offer%20a,source%20of%20long%2Dterm%20care. Accessed July 17, 2020.

29. Overview and Facts - NADSA: adult day services. NADSA: adult day services. Available at: https://www.nadsa.org/consumers/overview-and-facts/. Accessed July 17, 2020.

30. Adult day care. (2020). Available at: https://www.aginginplace.org/adult-day-care/. Accessed July 17, 2020.

31. Gaugler JE, Jarrott SE, Zarit SH, et al. Adult day service use and reductions in caregiving hours: effects on stress and psychological well-being for dementia caregivers. Int J Geriatr Psychiatry 2002;18(1):55–62.

32. Eng C, Pedulla J, Eleazer GP, et al. Program of all-inclusive care for the elderly (PACE): an innovative model of integrated geriatric care and financing. J Am Geriatr Soc 1997;45(2):223–32.

33. National Pace Association. (n.d.) Pace by the numbers. Retrieved 17 July, 2020. Available at: https://www.npaonline.org/sites/default/files/3186_pace_infographic_update_121819_combined_v1.pdf. Accessed July 14, 2020.

34. PACE Programs. Available at: https://pacenation.org/pace-programs/. Accessed July 14, 2019.

35. Keough ME, Fields TD, Gurwitz JH. A model of community-based interdisciplinary team training in the care of the frail elderly. Acad Med 2002;77(9):936.

36. Centers for Medicare and Medicade Services. Regulations and guidance. Available at: https://www.cms.gov/Regulations-and-Guidance/Guidance/Manuals/Downloads/pace111c06.pdf. Accessed July 14, 2020.

37. Oishi M. *A* national study of dental care delivery and utilization at programs of all-inclusive care for the elderly (PACE). Available at: https://ir.uiowa.edu/etd/6481/. Accessed July, 17 2020.
38. Mezey M, Mitty E, Burger SG. Nursing homes as a clinical site for training geriatric health care professionals. J Am Med Dir Assoc 2009;10(3):196–203.
39. Mueller CA, Tetzlaff B, Theile G, et al. Interprofesional collaboration and communication in nursing homes: a qualitative exploration of problems in medical care for nursing home residents- study protocol. J Adv Nurs 2014;71(2):451–7.
40. National Center for Biotechnology Information. Size and demographics of aging populations. Available at: https://www.ncbi.nlm.nih.gov/books/NBK51841/. Accessed July 17, 2020.
41. Porter J, Ntouva A, Read A, et al. The impact of oral health on the quality of life of nursing home residents. Health Qual Life Outcomes 2015;13(1). https://doi.org/10.1186/s12955-015-0300-y.
42. Family caregiver alliance. Selected long-term care statistics. Available at: https://www.caregiver.org/selected-long-term-care-statistics. Accessed July 17, 2020.
43. Avelino-Silva TJ, Jaluul O. Malnutrition in hospitalized older patients: management strategies to improve patient care and clinical outcomes. Int J Gerontol 2017;11(2):56–61.
44. Sheldon N. Home care industry grows to accommodate aging population. Rochester Business Journal 2018. Available at: https://rbj.net/2018/04/23/home-care-industry-grows-to-accommodate-aging-population/.
45. Spetz J, Trupin L, Bates T, et al. Future demand for long-term care workers will be influenced by demographic and utilization changes. Health Aff 2015;34(6): 936–45.
46. Palaganas JC, Epps C, Raemer DB. A history of simulation-enhanced interprofessional education. J Interprof Care 2013;28(2):110–5.
47. Pugh C, Kyle RR, Murray WB. Simulation and high-stakes testing. In: Clinical simulation: operations, engineering, and management. Burlington (VT): Elsevier Academic; 2008. p. 655.
48. Interprofessional education collaborative expert panel. Core competencies for interprofessional collaborative practice: report of an expert panel. Washington DC interprofessional education collaborative. Available at: https://nebula.wsimg.com/3ee8a4b5b5f7ab794c742b14601d5f23?AccessKeyId=DC06780E69ED19E2B3A5&disposition=0&alloworigin=1. Accessed July 17, 2020.
49. University California San Francisco. Program for interprofessional practice and education. Available at: https://interprofessional.ucsf.edu/our-approach. Accessed July 17, 2020.
50. University of Michigan. Interprofessional education. Available at: https://medicine.umich.edu/medschool/education/md-program/curriculum/longitudinal-learning/interprofessional-education. Accessed July 17, 2020.
51. Collins RJ, Friedman JW. The future of payment for dental care. Curr Oral Health Rep 2018;5:147–53.
52. American Dental Association. Supply and profile of dentists. Available at: https://www.ada.org/en/science-research/health-policy-institute/data-center/supply-and-profile-of-dentists. Accessed July, 17, 2020.

Innovations in Geriatric Oral Health Care

Elisa M. Ghezzi, DDS, PhD[a],*, Linda C. Niessen, DMD, MPH, MPP[b],
Judith A. Jones, DDS, MPH, DScD[c]

KEYWORDS

- Aging • Geriatric dental medicine • Innovations • Oral health care • Geriatrics

KEY POINTS

- Older adults are retaining their teeth and need strategies for a lifetime of oral health care.
- Innovations in geriatric oral health care must include integration of dental care with medical care, because older adults manifest multiple chronic conditions and take numerous medications that can affect oral health.
- Innovations in geriatric oral health care involve advances in clinical oral health care, delivery and models of care, funding, research, education, and policy.
- Daily prevention with interprofessional collaboration and professional preventive care have the most significant impacts on reducing oral disease in the aging population.

INTRODUCTION TO INNOVATIONS IN GERIATRIC ORAL HEALTH CARE

Baby boomers differ from their predecessors in many ways. Their active life expectancy has increased relative to their parents, and their aging is accompanied by their own unique needs, many differing from those of their parents. One major difference is that many baby boomers are retaining most of their teeth for their life span. This change has increased the need for dental care, especially preventive care. The impact of maintaining teeth for a lifetime also creates new challenges for nonsurgical and surgical dental treatment options. As patients, the baby boomers also bring comorbidities of medical conditions and medications that affect oral health. Providing oral health care where senior populations reside requires innovations affecting care delivery. Addressing these complexities requires looking beyond traditional dental care settings and treatment options, including a variety of collaborative efforts within and outside of the dental profession.

This article originally appeared in Dental Clinics, Volume 65 Issue 2, April 2021.
The authors have no conflict of interest.
[a] University of Michigan School of Dentistry, 26024 Pontiac Trail, South Lyon, MI 48178, USA;
[b] College of Dental Medicine, Kansas City University of Medicine and Biosciences, 2901 St. John's Boulevard, Joplin, MO 64804, USA; [c] University of Detroit Mercy School of Dentistry, 2700 Martin Luther King Jr. Boulevard, Room 401, Detroit, MI 48208-2576, USA
* Corresponding author.
E-mail address: eghezzi@umich.edu

Clin Geriatr Med 39 (2023) 343–357
https://doi.org/10.1016/j.cger.2023.01.005

The purpose of this article is to describe innovations that are transforming geriatric oral health and geriatric oral health care. Advances in clinical oral treatments are addressed as well as delivery and models of care, funding, research, education, and policy.

INNOVATIONS IN CLINICAL ORAL HEALTH CARE
Diagnosis and Treatment Planning

Clinical care begins with a comprehensive history, oral examination, radiographic imaging, and diagnostic tests, depending on a patient's chief complaint. Radiographic imaging has seen advances with the use of the cone beam computer tomography (CBCT) in dentistry. CBCT is used most frequently for diagnosis and treatment in endodontics, implants, and oral surgery. For patients who are wheelchair bound, portable radiographic systems are available. In addition, when clinicians are using a portable radiographic system or taking radiographs for patients who are in wheelchairs, the extension cone paralleling radiographic positioning system, although not new, helps ensure that the radiographs taken are positioned correctly.

Once a patient's history and physical are taken and radiographic imaging completed, it is important to document findings in the patient's record. The electronic health record (EHR) can facilitate the recording of the patient's information and the integration of the patient's dental with medical findings. Most dental EHRs do not interface with medical EHRs. To the extent that future dental EHRs become part of a patient's medical record or can bridge with the patient's medical record, the patient's physician and dentist will be able to coordinate care better, in a more seamless manner.

Preventive Oral Health Care

Because baby boomers retain more teeth, they continue to suffer from preventable oral diseases. With increased comorbidities, such as chronic diseases and medication usage, both the need for and value of preventive oral health care increase. In addition, ageist stereotypes continue to promulgate the belief that poor oral health and tooth loss are a natural part of the aging process. Older adults do not lose teeth because they have an eightieth birthday; they lose teeth because they have dental diseases that can be prevented.

Older adults continue to be at risk for not only tooth-related diseases, such as coronal caries, root caries, and periodontal disease, but also various oral lesions, such as oral candidiasis and oral cancer. Thus, regular visits for dental examinations and preventive oral health care are critically important to successful aging by decreasing oral inflammation and maintaining overall health and oral health.

Daily home care is the first step in a successful oral care preventive program. If an older adult has medical diseases that inhibit the ability to provide self-care, such as a stroke, dementia, or severe rheumatoid arthritis, caregiver assistance may be required. For some patients, the most effective prophylaxis may occur in the dental office.

Preventive oral care in the dental office begins with the dental team conducting a risk assessment for oral diseases on each patient. If an older adult smokes and takes multiple medications, the risk for root caries, periodontal disease, and/or oral cancer all may be elevated. Caries risk assessment forms are available from the American Dental Association (ADA).[1] In 2013, the ADA provided clinical recommendations for the use of topical fluorides in adults.[2] Based on the literature review and consensus, the recommendations provide for professionally applied or prescription-strength home-use topical fluorides for patients at high caries risk. These include professionally applied 2.26% fluoride varnish or 1.23% acidulated phosphate fluoride gel. For home use, the recommendations included a 5000–parts per million (ppm) (0.5%) fluoride prescription strength home use gel or paste or 0.09% fluoride mouth rinse.

Once risk levels are identified, the dental team can implement new preventive technologies to lower an individual's risk. Topical fluorides and fluoride varnishes have been shown to be effective in adults as well as children.[2] Silver diamine fluoride (SDF), a new topical fluoride application, which has been used to prevent caries in children, now is being used to control root caries in older adults. A 2018 systematic review examined SDF applied to exposed root surfaces to control root caries.[3] The investigators included only studies with a 12-month follow-up. The review found that SDF applications performed better than the placebo in preventing root caries. SDF was as effective as chlorhexidine or sodium fluoride varnish. The investigators suggested that 38% SDF applications once a year to exposed root surfaces "are simple, inexpensive and effective way" to prevent root caries. They also noted that the complaints about the black staining of the carious lesions caused by SDF "were rare among older adults."

A disadvantage of the use of SDF is black staining of the tooth. If caries is present on the coronal or root surface, applying SDF causes the tooth to stain black. For some older adults, this side effect could be unacceptable. It is important for patients to be informed of this side effect and provide informed consent.

Fluoride varnishes and SDF along with 5000-ppm daily fluoride toothpaste provide important options to prevent caries in high-risk patients. An aggressive approach to preventing caries is warranted for patients with various medical conditions, particularly patients who suffer from a dry mouth or patients who are unable to cooperate with traditional restorative dental treatment.

Minimally Invasive Restorative Care

Like surgery in general, the trend in the management of dental caries has become more minimally invasive. In the past, recurrent caries was treated by removing the entire restoration and replacing it. Today, with greater understanding of the caries process, if recurrent caries is detected, it is recommended to remove the caries only. If the caries does not undermine the restoration, replace only that portion of the restoration affected by the recurrent caries.[4]

Minimally invasive therapy for the treatment of root caries has been described by Dr Jane Chalmers[5] at the University of Iowa, who advocated removing the caries using a round bur on a low-speed handpiece. The resulting preparation is conservative, having not removed any unnecessary hard tissue. Once the caries is removed, the operator can assess the surgical field for moisture control and then determine which restorative material to use to restore the tooth.[5] If a dry field can be maintained, then a composite resin can be placed. For patients who are unable to cooperate with restorative treatment and/or for whom moisture control is very difficult, fewer options are available for restoring the tooth, such as glass ionomers or silver amalgam.

Innovations in restorative materials center around bioactive materials. The mechanism of action for bioactivity varies by material. Some materials, such as glass ionomers, release fluoride and, thus, remineralize tooth structure. Other materials deposit hydroxyapatite, such as calcium aluminates. These materials also remineralize tooth structure. Newer materials being developed stimulate pulpal regeneration. These materials, primarily calcium silicates, such as mineral trioxide aggregate (MTA), can both remineralize and deposit hydroxyapatite. MTA is used most frequently in endodontic therapy.

Endodontic Therapy

As older adults retain teeth, there is a greater likelihood that they need endodontic therapy. A study by the American Board of Endodontics of its diplomats found that 26% of their patients were over age 65.[6] Because older adults may have more increased calcifications in the root canals, imaging is critical to the diagnosis and success of root canal therapy. Recently, CBCT has been used more commonly in endodontic treatment and has been shown to be effective in diagnosing various endodontic problems.[7]

The use of magnification and smaller files can assist in identifying and instrumenting calcified canals. Nickel titanium rotary instruments can increase the efficiency of root canal therapy compared with hand instruments, thus enabling a shorter appointment for the older patient.[8]

Older adults also can experience root fractures in restored or endodontically treated teeth. MTA is a bioactive endodontic cement that has been used in vital pulp therapy, for root perforations, to treat both vertical and horizontal fractures and in preserving teeth that in the past may have been extracted.[9–11] Innovations in bioactive endodontic cements continue and now offer patients with endodontically diseased teeth more options for treatment and retention of their teeth.

Implants

When older adults lose teeth, they can be replaced with dental implants to retain dentures or an implant-supported prosthesis. Although implants are more costly than traditional fixed and removable prostheses, for many patients, implants have become a more desirable treatment option because of their esthetics and function.[12] A 2018 study examining the prevalence of implants from 1999 to 2000 through 2015 to 2016 found that the 65-year-old to 74-year-old population had the largest absolute increase in implants use from 2000 to 2016 and the largest relative increase in prevalence of implants in 55-year-old to 64-year-old adults.[13] Although implant prevalence is low, the study showed that implant prevalence was increasing in older adults and is expected to continue to increase. The study also found that implant prevalence was higher in older adults with higher levels of education and more "advantaged groups."[13]

Although older adults may have more chronic diseases than younger adults, general health problems that contraindicate implant surgery are rare.[14] An historical prospective study examined implant survival in a cohort of patients born prior to 1950 who received dental implants in a single private dental office.[15] This study evaluated implant survival and success in an elderly population. It also assessed indicators and risk factors for success or failure of dental implants in older adults (ages 60 years and older). The study found that implants can be placed successfully in older adults. A variety of factors affect long-term success. One finding identified that implants that were placed where bone augmentation was performed before or during surgery did not have the same longevity as implants placed that did not require bone augmentation.[15]

Innovations in implant treatment continue. A minimally invasive approach and a digital workflow are revolutionizing the ease and efficiency of implant treatment of patients. The digital workflow with CBCT imaging is making the diagnosis and planning for the implant prosthesis much more convenient for patients, in addition to facilitating communication among the general dentist, specialist, and the dental laboratory. A minimally invasive approach to implant surgery is resulting in a decreased number of implants being placed to support a prosthesis. The sizes of the implants placed also are becoming smaller, shifting from standard diameter implants to more narrow diameter implants (or mini-implants). Mini-implants can reduce the need for bone augmentation and reduce complications associated with implant placement. Digital technologies and workflows will continue to advance the ease with which implant surgery and prostheses are planned and designed.

INNOVATIONS IN MODELS OF CARE TO IMPROVE ACCESS TO CARE
Daily Oral Care

As older adults are retaining their teeth for their lifetime, there has been a cultural shift from the expectation that people lose teeth as they age to an expectation that teeth will be kept. This marker of successful aging, however, requires an educational shift from denture care to an understanding that daily oral health care and prevention are critical to the maintenance of dentition. Education, communication, and resources are necessary to achieve this goal.

A priority for persons as they age is to maintain their autonomy. To the extent that a person can provide self-care, it is preferred. If and when cognitive and physical challenges arise and dependency on others increases, however, it becomes necessary for others to participate in the daily oral hygiene care. Autonomy should not be a priority to the detriment of appropriate care. Daily oral care assessment should be made to determine if the current level of care is appropriate or if further intervention is required.[16] These interventions could progress from verbal reminders to handing a toothbrush with toothpaste on it to complete toothbrushing and interdental cleaning by the caregiver.

There still exists significant need for education of family and professional caregivers to understand their critical role as evaluator and intervener. It is not uncommon for a family member's concern about halitosis to be resolved when they become aware of a removable partial denture that had not been removed and cleaned daily. Persons unable to perform activities of daily living independently need others to provide oral health care supplies and assess feasibility to sink access. Innovative educational Web sites and videos, such as Mouth Care without a Battle (http://www.mouthcarewithoutabattle.org/), have been produced to facilitate education of caregivers to provide oral health care for those with physical and/or behavioral challenges. Financial and transportation barriers can hinder the ability to purchase oral health care supplies. Innovative programs include providing toothbrushes, toothpaste, and interdental cleaners through Meals on Wheels program donations.

Professional Oral Health Care

Typically, professional oral health care is obtained at a dental office by a dental team composed of dentists, dental hygienists, and dental assistants. Wheelchair-bound patients often require assistance to transfer to the dental chair or need a transfer device, such as a Hoyer lift. For older adults who cannot be transported to a dental office, innovative delivery systems have been developed to provide mobile services in home and at long-term care (LTC) facilities. Mobile care can be provided in an equipped van or by equipment set up in an available room on location. These unique environments use innovative transportable equipment, such as handheld radiograph machines and portable dental operatories complete with compressors.

Collaborative hygiene practice has expanded the ability of dental hygienists to provide preventive oral health care in LTC settings without a dentist present. Dental therapists are other dental providers licensed in some states with an expanded scope of duties, which enhance access to care for those in need of mobile dental services.

Although both of these innovative practice models of care have expanded access to care in many states, the benefit has not been fully realized due to limited training, restrictive regulations, and minimal financial incentives.

Teledentistry

The virtual dental home is an innovation that has improved access to care for patients with limited mobility and access to care. It is "based on the principles of bringing care to places where underserved populations live, work or receive social, educational or general health services, integrating oral health with general health, social, and educational delivery systems. Using telehealth technologies to connect a geographically distributed, collaborative dental team with the dentist at the head of team-making decisions about treatment and location of services is paramount."[17] Teledentistry is evolving to enhance triage assessment often used in collaborative care settings when a dentist is not present for treatment.

The 2019 coronavirus disease (COVID-19) pandemic created an explosion in teledentistry with the inability of oral health providers to have in-person contact with patients, especially those residing in LTC settings. Teledentistry can be used when dental professionals are distant (off site) from patients to evaluate and suggest modifications to daily oral health care as well as troubleshoot other oral pathology issues, such as concerns about a dental abscess or a burning mouth. Missing fillings, presence of tori, denture sores, and retained roots can be triaged by assessing the level of urgency for care, determining an acute need for immediate care or chronic condition requiring observation. Treatment considerations include prescriptions (eg, antibiotics, antifungals, fluoride), referral to an outside provider, on-site treatment, and continued observation.

Educational training in teledentistry for the health care team includes all LTC staff from medical directors to nursing assistants and requires access and competency in digital technologies. Teledentistry in LTC facilities is underutilized where the dental providers and the health care teams have limited access to protocols (Health Insurance Portability and Accountability Act compliance, consent, and so forth), equipment, or experience. Lack of educational training in teledentistry due to cost (eg, minimal to no reimbursement), limited time (eg, competing priorities), and limited access to oral health care trainers jeopardizes the ability to identify oral health issues requiring attention. Webinars sponsored by aging and oral health organizations are being developed to enhance knowledge and interest in this area.

Interprofessional Collaborative Care in Long-Term Care

Given the complicated clinical conditions of older adults, dental providers need to collaborate with other health care providers in the assessment of the geriatric patient. Nationally recognized programs, such as the Oral Health Nursing Education and Practice Program (OHNEP) (http://ohnep.org/), are increasing interprofessional education across disciplines by including oral health in assessment tools (head, eyes, ears, nose, oral cavity, and throat [HEENOT] examination). An oral component should be included in annual history and physical examinations by all health care providers. Health care teams need to understand oral health conditions and disease processes, thereby becoming knowledgeable about what precipitates a need for immediate intervention versus oral disease that can be attentively observed. Smiles for Life (www.smilesforlifeoralhealth.org), a national oral health curriculum designed to enhance the role of primary care clinicians in the promotion of oral health, has a module dedicated to geriatric oral health. Practical guidelines for physicians in promoting oral health in frail older adults are being developed to educate and provide clinical directives to health care providers beyond the dental team.[18] Dental professionals can learn from medical and nursing teams how to manage behavioral and cognitive challenges, just as medical and nursing teams can learn oral pathology from dental professionals.

Typically, daily oral hygiene care in the LTC setting is the responsibility of certified nursing assistants, who should be trained not only on oral hygiene techniques but also on how to provide an oral assessment, with clear guidelines to trigger appropriate referral, and on required personal protective equipment. Largely due to lack of reimbursement, the role of the registered dental hygienist in the management of oral health care in LTC settings has been woefully underutilized. The dental hygienist is capable of assessing and documenting residents' oral status, managing daily oral care, educating the LTC staff, providing routine professional care, and making referrals as needed.

Interprofessional collaboration initiatives in LTC need to provide sustainable oral health care for residents, especially when oral health care providers are not accessible. The COVID-19 pandemic created a critical opportunity for education of providers (eg, medical directors, health care providers, and caregivers) for assessments with use of pictures to provide dental professionals with information necessary to address oral hygiene, dental problems, and necessary referrals. Since the coronavirus pandemic, the use of video conferencing meetings has become a way of conducting daily business. A video meeting can serve as a means to conduct in-service education for the LTC team, with dental professionals showing clinical photographs of common conditions and answering LTC team questions. The pandemic also highlighted the need for an evidence-based approach to providing oral health care for patients throughout their life.

Oral Health Care Paradigms

A need for a structured, evidence-based approach to care for older adults resulted in the development of the Seattle Care Pathways.[19] As patients transition from robust to complete dependency, the model guides oral health care providers, detailing assessment, treatment planning, prevention, and communication. As dependency levels increase, goals change from comprehensive care to care focused on comfort, prevention, dignity, and safety.[20]

Treatment planning for the aging patient must be individually based and enhance their quality of life.[21] The rational treatment plan includes evaluation of numerous factors that affect both the patient and the dentist's ability to provide care. These factors include the patient's desires and expectations, the type and severity of the patient's dental needs, how the patient's dental problems affect quality of life, the patient's ability to tolerate the stress of treatment, the patient's ability to maintain oral health independently, the probability of positive treatment outcomes, the availability of reasonable and less-extensive treatment alternatives, the patient's financial status, the dentist's ability to deliver the care needed (eg, resources, skills, and equipment), and other issues (eg, the patient's life span, family influences and expectations, and bioethical issues).[22]

Models of Care Integrating Medicine and Dental Medicine

There are several innovative care models for older adults in the United States. The Administration for Community Living project (https://oralhealth.acl.gov) online database of community-based oral health programs assists state and local level groups in starting or enhancing oral health programs for older adults. A Community Guide to Adult Oral Health Program Implementation is a toolkit for community-based entities to find key tips, case studies, interactive tools, and other sources of support for creating cost-effective, sustainable programs.

Dental clinics in community health centers and federally qualified health centers often are physically located in a separate clinic but have collaborative relationships with the other medical disciplines housed under the same roof. Interdisciplinary clinics provide dental professionals with automatic referrals for medical care. The Geriatric Research, Education, and Clinical Centers in the Veterans Affairs Medical Centers (VAMCs) have a long-standing model of interprofessional care. In addition to VAMCs, other fully integrated systems of care that share medical and dental records include Programs of All-Inclusive Care for the Elderly (PACE), Kaiser Permanente, and Health Partners.[23]

INNOVATIONS IN FUNDING MODELS
Value-Based Models

New funding models are being evaluated for application to dentistry for older adults. For example, value-based care is being considered. Value in oral health care can be defined as quality/cost. Applied to oral health care, *value* aims to prevent rather than react to disease. For example, if a measure of quality is a dental visit once or twice a year, that measure of quality (visit) is divided by cost. Similarly, if a person is at high risk for dental caries, as defined by 1 or 2 new carious lesions that need treatment per year, the value of preventive treatment is the quality (fluoride treatments) divided by the cost. Tooth retention could be another measure. The Japanese 80/20 Movement promoted keeping 20 or more natural teeth by the age of 80 because tooth retention was an indicator for reduced medical expenses.[24] If the percent of 80-year-old adults with 20 or more teeth increases, the percent of the population with adequate tooth retention/cost could be measured.

Inclusion of Dental Care in Medicare Part B

A large and growing number of organizations, including the Gerontological Society of America (https://www.geron.org/), American Association of Retired Persons (https://www.aarp.org/), the Santa Fe Group (https://santafegroup.org/) and the Center for Medicare Advocacy (https://medicareadvocacy.org/) have policies that support the inclusion of a dental benefit in Medicare. Measures to include a basic and expanded benefit have been described.[25] Premium costs are estimated to be $32 per person per month for a basic benefit, and an optional $32 per month for more extensive benefits.[25]

Volunteer Programs

Programs like the Volunteer for Dental (https://volunteerdental.org/) offer free dental care in exchange for volunteer service in local communities. The program in Muskegon, Michigan, offers free screening, basic dental care, referrals to dentists for additional services, oral health education, and community events in exchange for community volunteering.

Discount Programs

Some insurance companies and dentists in private practice offer discount card programs for those without dental insurance, providing reduced cost of care for participation or membership in the program. In addition, dental hygiene and dental schools offer moderately discounted services for the entire community; however, patients in educational institutions must be prepared to spend more time in the dental chair. Fortunately, these services are well supervised, with students undergoing strict evaluations of the care they provide in a learning environment.

INNOVATIONS IN RESEARCH

Research has demonstrated the clear association between oral and systemic diseases, and findings in this area continue to strengthen.

Type 2 Diabetes Mellitus

Type 2 diabetes mellitus and periodontal diseases have a clear 2-way link.[26–29] People with type 2 diabetes mellitus are more likely to develop periodontal disease, and the presence of periodontal disease interferes with the control of diabetes. Although research suggests periodontal treatment can decrease systemic inflammation, allowing for better glycemic control,[30] further research will help clarify this relationship.

Cardiovascular Disease

The oral inflammation present in periodontal diseases is considered an independent risk factor for coronary heart disease, increasing risk by 24% to 35%.[31] The number of teeth remaining also is significantly associated with fatal and nonfatal myocardial infarctions. Myocardial infarctions are associated with low-grade chronic inflammation.[32] Research has yet to confirm, however, that treatment of periodontal disease improves cardiovascular outcomes.[31,33]

Rheumatoid Arthritis

Bacterial antigens found in the periodontium and gastrointestinal tract may contribute to the etiology of rheumatoid arthritis.[34] Studies show an association between rheumatoid arthritis and complete tooth loss as well as periodontal disease.[35,36]

Tooth Loss and Cognition

Recent studies suggest that oral diseases and tooth loss are associated with dementia.[37–39] Nilsson and colleagues[40] showed a positive association between tooth loss, periodontal bone loss, and cognitive function. A longitudinal cohort study among South Korean older adults reported an association of early-state cognitive impairment with increases in tooth loss.[41] Importantly, not all of the current studies control for education, income, smoking, self-reported health, and health status.

Independent of the number of teeth present, a 2019 study in *Science Advances* demonstrated that the bacterium, *Porphyromonas gingivalis,* a periodontal pathogen, was present in the brains of patients with Alzheimer disease. *P gingivalis* produces toxic proteases called gingipains, which also were found in the brains of Alzheimer patients and cause pathology to the tau proteins in the brain. This finding provided evidence for causation of Alzheimer's disease and a rationale for treatment with small molecule gingipain inhibitors to prevent neurodegeneration.[42]

Several systematic reviews also are available. Cerutti-Kopplin and colleagues)[43] conducted a systematic review (n = 10 studies) and meta-analysis (n = 8 studies) that showed that persons with a suboptimal dentition (<20 teeth) had a higher risk for developing cognitive decline (HR 1.26; 95% CI, 1.14–1.40) than persons with greater than 20 teeth. Chen and colleagues'[44] meta-analysis of 8 cohort studies reported that tooth loss was associated with a 1.3- times greater risk of developing dementia with an increase of number of teeth lost. Oh and colleagues[45] conducted a systematic review and meta-analysis of 11 cohort studies; they suggest that having more teeth is associated with an almost 50% lower risk of dementia. Oh and colleagues, however, rated the quality of the evidence as very low.

In the other direction, declines in cognitive function are associated with poor oral conditions. Foley and colleagues[46] conducted a meta-analysis of 28 studies that examined the oral health status of persons with dementia; they found that across a variety of oral health measures (tooth loss, oral hygiene, dental caries, and so forth), persons with dementia had worse oral health. Furthermore, work by Naorungroj and colleagues,[47] using data on cognitive function and oral health status in the Atherosclerosis Risk in Communities study, suggest that before even before dementia becomes apparent, cognitive decline may contribute to deterioration in oral health as measured by oral hygiene and tooth loss. Given the devastation of cognitive decline on individuals and families and the human and financial costs to society, further research on the association of tooth loss, oral diseases, and cognition is needed.

INNOVATIONS IN EDUCATION

Geriatric dental medicine in the United Kingdom and Australia is considered a specialty of dentistry. With specialty status comes advanced education programs in the field. Both the United Kingdom and Australia have seen research advance in the field of geriatric dental medicine along with funding to support these efforts. Although diplomate status exists for geriatric dental medicine (and hospital dentistry) conducted by Special Care in Dentistry, it is not recognized as a specialty by the ADA National Commission on Recognition of Specialties. To achieve this, geriatric dental medicine would need to develop criteria for advanced education programs in geriatric dental medicine and have these programs accredited by the Commission on Dental Accreditation. The organization, Special Care in Dentistry, has had discussions among its members about working toward the development of geriatric dental medicine and/or special needs dentistry as a specialty in the United States. It is not clear when this will occur.

With the lack of specialty status, dentists interested in learning more about geriatric dental medicine often pursue advanced education in general dentistry. A few geriatric dental fellowships continue to educate dentists in formal 1-year to 2-year programs. These programs focus on understanding the differences between age-associated changes and disease-associated changes in health and oral health. Clinical components of the program often focus on providing dental care to medically complex patients in outpatient settings, in LTC or assisted-living facilities, or using mobile or portable dental equipment. Because the number of advanced education programs in geriatric dental medicine is limited, most dentists interested in learning more about geriatric dental medicine attend short-term continuing education programs.

Dental hygienists, dental therapists, and expanded function hygienists have even fewer formal programs available to them in geriatric dental medicine. Many learn through continuing education courses and on-the-job education, working with a mentor in geriatric dental medicine.

Nowhere is the need for integration of medicine and dental medicine greater than in the geriatric patients. For dentists, it is critical to understand the medical history and medications the patient is taking, along with the social factors that affect a patient's ability to get to the dental office, daily hygiene care, and so forth. Similarly, it is critical for physician, nursing, and pharmacy colleagues to have a basic understanding of oral health and disease to make referrals to dental professionals as needed. In LTC facilities, often dental hygienists and dentists are invited to provide in-service continuing education to the nursing and medical staff. These interprofessional oral health education opportunities will continue to increase in importance as the older population increases.

Finally, as the population ages, consumers continue to be interested in learning more about health, including oral health. Social media and health Web sites serve as sources of information about oral health, with some much more reputable than others. Reputable sources, such as the ADA and the National Institute for Dental and Craniofacial Research at the National Institutes of Health, have developed Web sites, Mouthhealthy.org and https://www.nidcr.nih.gov/health-info/for-older-adults, that provide information for consumers on oral health. Various disease-specific Web sites for older adults, such as the Alzheimer's Association, provides information pro-vide information on oral health for adults with dementia. "Tooth Wisdom: Get Smart About Your Mouth" is a seminar series developed for seniors to provide information about oral health and how to maintain it.

INNOVATIONS IN POLICY AND COLLABORATION

The Fédération Dentaire International (World Dental Federation) developed a toolkit for healthy aging based on the principles of providing for the oral health care needs to today's older adults, reinforcing prevention activities throughout the life-course, and adapting health systems to set up evidence-based prevention and care strate-gies.[48] Eight core pillars were identified: (1) integration of oral care into general care; (2) promotion of oral health throughout the life-course; (3) shaping of

---

Box 1
Future directions for innovations in geriatric oral health care

Oral health policy
  Establish dental benefit in Medicare.
  National health organizations: establish policies to enhance importance of oral health for
    the aging and develop guidelines for policy and direction for research.
  National health authorities: develop policies, funding, measurable goals, and targets for oral
    health for the aging, including mandates for services in LTC facilities.
  Local coalitions and community organizations: develop collaborative partnerships with
    stakeholders and promote the implementation of policies that support evidence-based
    strategies to provide optimal oral health for the aging.

Oral health care
  National public health programs: incorporate oral health promotion and disease prevention
    based on a common risk factor approach.
  Investigate alternative models through mobile dentistry, telemedicine, and home care to
    improve access to professional oral health care for the aging.
  Enhance access to preventive daily oral care for the aging through trained caregivers.

Education and training
  Develop a specialty in geriatric dental medicine.
  Create interdisciplinary collaboration and training with health care teams and caregivers.
  Establish oral health care resources for providers of care for the aging targeting the patient,
    family, and caregivers.
  Address workforce shortage through training program funding, enhanced training of oral
    health care professionals in the care of the aging, and alternative workforce models.

Research
  Provide outcomes of oral health intervention programs and workforce models for policy
    development.
  Include oral health for the aging as a component of aging and chronic disease research.
  Investigate whether improvement of oral conditions will decrease cognitive decline.
  Examine the longitudinal impact of improving oral conditions on noncommunicable diseases
    (cardiovascular disease, type 2 diabetes mellitus, hypertension, and stroke).

Adapted from Ghezzi EM, Kobayashi K, Park DY, Srisilapanan P. Oral healthcare systems for an ageing population: concepts and challenges. International Dental Journal 67(Suppl. 2): 26-33; 2017.

evidence-based oral health policies; (4) removal of financial barriers; (5) removal of physical barriers; (6) provision of appropriate oral health care; (7) mobilization of all stakeholders along the care pathways; and (8) fostering of community-based programs.

The Santa Fe Group (http://santafegroup.org/) has led efforts in research and advocacy convening a coalition of stakeholders from dentistry, aging, health care, and industry in support of Medicare coverage for medically necessary oral and dental health therapies. From this work, the Medicare Oral Health Coalition has been established by Families USA (https://familiesusa.org/).

The Gerontological Society of America[49] published a white paper on interprofessional solutions for improving oral health in older adults, addressing access barriers, and creating oral health champions by identifying the need for interprofessional education and practice, promotion of an oral health benefit in Medicare, and creation of coalitions and oral health champions for health promotion and public awareness campaigns while providing practical calls to action. An example is the Coalition for Oral Health for the Aging (https://www.micoha.org/), which works nationally (1) to be a resource for providers of care for the aging; (2) to promote the implementation of policies that support evidence-based strategies that provide optimal oral health for the aging; and (3) to develop collaborative partnerships that address the oral health needs of the aging.[50]

SUMMARY

Future innovations in geriatric oral health care (**Box 1**) must address oral health policy, care, education, training, and research. Only a life course approach will allow achieving the ultimate goal, to increase the number and percent of elders who maintain their natural teeth and oral health for a lifetime. This life course approach must be interprofessional and integrate dental care with medical care. For elders to age successfully, they must maintain health and function throughout their lives. Traditional dental professionals and delivery systems must be expanded. There is no way to predict what the next advancements in technology will bring what they will allow accomplishing.

CLINICS CARE POINTS

- The COVID-19 pandemic created an explosion in teledentistry, with the inability of oral health providers to have in-person contact with patients, especially those residing in LTC settings.
- Daily prevention with interprofessional collaboration should include toothbrushing with a fluoride toothpaste as well as prescription-strength topical fluoride application.
- Professional preventive care includes not only regular dental cleanings but also application of fluoride varnish to reduce decay.
- SDF is a novel and effective treatment to reduce progression of decay, especially for those older adults with difficulty in cooperating with dental treatment.

REFERENCES

1. American Dental Association. Caries risk assessment form >6 years 2020. Available at: ADA.org. Accessed July 22, 2020.

2. American Dental Association. Clinical recommendations for topical fluorides. 2013. Available at: ADA.org. Accessed July 22, 2020.
3. Oliveira BH, Cunha-Cruz J, Rajendra A, et al. Controlling caries in exposed root surface with silver diamine fluoride:a systematic review with meta-analyses. JADA 2018;149(8):671–9.
4. Kidd EAM. Essentials of dental caries: the disease and its management. 3rd edition. New York: Oxford University Press, Inc; 2005. p. 190.
5. Chalmers JM. Minimal intervention dentistry: part 2. Strategies for addressing restorative challenges in older patients. J Can Dent Assoc 2006;72(5):435–40.
6. Goodis HE, Rossall JC, Kahn AJ. Endodontic status in older US adults. Report of a survey. JADA 2001;132:1525–30.
7. Venskutonis T, Plotino G, Juodzbalys G, et al. The importance of cone-beam computed tomography in the management of endodontic problems: a review of the literature. J Endod 2014;40(12):1895–901.
8. Guelzow A, Stamm O, Martus P, et al. Comparative study of six rotary nickel-titanium systems and hand instrumentation for root canal preparation. Int Endod J 2005;38:743–52.
9. Parirokh M, Torabinejad M, Dummer PMH. Mineral trioxide aggregate and other bioactive endodontic cements: an updated overview - part I: vital pulp therapy. Int Endod J 2018;51(2):177–205.
10. Parirokh M, Torabinejad M. Mineral trioxide aggregate: a comprehensive literature review–Part III: Clinical applications, drawbacks, and mechanism of action. J Endod 2010;36(3):400–13.
11. Bakland LK, Andreasen JO. Will mineral trioxide aggregate replace calcium hydroxide in treating pulpal and periodontal healing complications subsequent to dental trauma? A review. Dent Traumatol 2012;2012(1):25–32.
12. Tarnow DP. Commentary: replacing missing teeth with dental implants. A century of progress. J Periodontol 2014;85(11):1475–7.
13. Elani HW, Starr JR, DaSilva JD, et al. Trends in Dental Implant Use in the US 1999-2016 and Projections to 2026. J Dent Res 2018;97(13):1424–30.
14. Renouard F, Rangert B. Risk factors in implant dentistry: simplified clinical analysis for predictable treatment. 2nd edition. Paris: Quintessence International; 2008. p. 1–18.
15. Compton SM, Clark D, Chan S, et al. Dental implants in the elderly population: a long-term follow-up. Int J Oral Maxillofac Implants 2017;32(1):164–70.
16. Ghezzi EM, Fisher MM. Strategies for oral health care practitioners to manage older adults through care-setting transitions. J Calif Dent Assoc 2019;47(4): 235–45.
17. Glassman P. Virtual dental home. J Calif Dent Assoc 2012;40(7):564–6.
18. Kossioni AE, Hajto-Bryk J, Janssens B, et al. Practical guidelines for physicians in promoting oral health in frail older adults. J Am Med Directors Assoc 2018;19(12): 1039–46.
19. Pretty IA, Ellwood RP, Lo ECM, et al. The Seattle Care Pathway for securing oral health in older patients. Gerodontology 2014;31(Suppl 1):77–87.
20. Jones JA, Brown EJ, Volicer L. Target outcomes for long-term oral health care in dementia: a Delphi approach. J Public Health Dent 2000;60(4):330–4.
21. Ettinger RL. Treatment planning concepts for the ageing patient. Aust Dent J 2015;60(Suppl 1):71–85.
22. Lindquist TJ, Ettinger RL. The complexities involved with managing the care of an elderly patient. J Am Dent Assoc 2003;134(5):593–600.

23. Jones JA, Snyder JJ, Gesko DS, et al. Integrated medical-dental delivery systems: models in a changing environment and their implications for dental education. J Dent Educ 2017;81(9):eS21–9.

24. Shinsho F. New strategy for better geriatric oral health in Japan: 80/20 Movement and Healthy Japan 21. Int Dental J 2001;51(3 Suppl):200–6.

25. Jones JA, Monopoli M. Designing a new payment model for oral care for seniors. Compendium 2017;38(9):622–9.

26. Chapple IL, Genco R, working group 2 of the joint EFP/AAP workshop. Diabetes and periodontal diseases: consensus report of the Joint EFP/AAP Workshop on Periodontitis and Systemic Diseases. J Periodontol 2013;84(4 Suppl):S106–12.

27. Genco RJ, Borgnakke WS. Diabetes as a potential risk for periodontitis: association studies. Periodontol 2000 2020;83(1):40–5.

28. Genco RJ, Graziani F, Hasturk H. Effects of periodontal disease on glycemic control, complications, and incidence of diabetes mellitus. Periodontol 2000 2020; 83(1):59–65.

29. Genco RJ, Grossi SG, Ho A, et al. A proposed model linking inflammation to obesity, diabetes, and periodontal infections. J Periodontol 2005;76(Suppl 11S):2075–84.

30. Kudiyirickal MG, Pappachan JM. Diabetes Mellitus and Oral Health. Endocrine 2015;49(1):27–34.

31. Humphrey LL, Fu R, Buckley DI, et al. Periodontal disease and coronary heart disease incidence: a systematic review and meta-analysis. J Gen Intern Med 2008;23(12):2079–86.

32. Holmlund A, Lampa E, Lind L. Oral health and cardiovascular disease risk in a cohort of periodontitis patients. Atherosclerosis 2017;262:101–6.

33. Li C, Lv Z, Shi Z, et al. Periodontal therapy for the management of cardiovascular disease in patients with chronic periodontitis. Cochrane Database Syst Rev 2017; 11(11):CD009197.

34. Nikitakis NG, Papaioannou W, Sakkas LI, et al. The autoimmunity-oral microbiome connection. Oral Dis 2017;23(7):828–39.

35. Bender P, Burgin WB, Sculean A, et al. Serum antibody levels against *Porphyromonas gingivalis* in patients with and without rheumatoid arthritis - a systematic review and meta-analysis. Clin Oral Investig 2017;21(1):33–42.

36. Felton DA. Complete Edentulism and Comorbid Diseases: An Update. J Prosthodont 2016;25(1):5–20.

37. Fang WL, Jiang MJ, Gu BB, et al. Tooth loss as a risk factor for dementia: systematic review and meta-analysis of 21 observational studies. BMC Psychiatry 2018; 18(1):345.

38. Han SH, Wu B, Burr JA. Edentulism and Trajectories of Cognitive Functioning Among Older Adults: The Role of Dental Care Service Utilization. J Aging Health 2019. https://doi.org/10.1177/0898264319851654.

39. Saito S, Ohi T, Murakami T, et al. Association between tooth loss and cognitive impairment in community-dwelling older Japanese adults: a 4-year prospective cohort study from the Ohasama study. BMC Oral Health 2018;18:142.

40. Nilsson H, Berglund JS, Renvert S. Periodontitis, tooth loss and cognitive functions among older adults. Clin Oral Investig 2018;22(5):2103–9.

41. Yoo JJ, Yoon JH, Kang MJ, et al. The effect of missing teeth on dementia in older people: a nationwide population-based cohort study in South Korea. BMC Oral Health 2019;19(1):61.

42. Dominy SS, Lynch C, Ermini F, et al. *Porphyromonas gingivalis* in Alzheimer's disease brains: Evidence for disease causation and treatment with small-molecule inhibitors. Sci Adv 2019;5:1–21.
43. Cerutti-Kopplin D, Feine J, Padilha DM, et al. Tooth loss increases the risk of diminished cognitive function: a systematic review and meta-analysis. JDR Clin Trans Res 2016;1(1):10–9.
44. Chen J, Ren CJ, Wu L, et al. Tooth loss is associated with increased risk of dementia and with a dose-response relationship. Front Aging Neurosci 2018; 10:415.
45. Oh B, Han DH, Han KT, et al. Association between residual teeth number in later life and incidence of dementia: a systematic review and meta-analysis. BMC Geriatr 2018;18(1):48.
46. Foley NC, Affoo RH, Siqueira WL, et al. A systematic review examining the oral health status of persons with dementia. JDR Clin Trans Res 2017;2(4):330–42.
47. Naorungroj S, Slade GD, Beck JD, et al. Cognitive decline and oral health in middle-aged adults in the ARIC study. J Dent Res 2013;92(9):795–801.
48. World Dental Federation FDI. Achieving a healthy ageing society 2018. Available at: https://www.fdiworlddental.org/sites/default/files/media/resources/ohap-2018-advocacy_doc-achieving_healthy_ageing_society.pdf. Accessed July 22, 2020.
49. The Gerontological Society of America. White paper on oral health: an Essential Element of health aging 2017. Available at: https://www.geron.org/images/gsa/documents/gsa2017oralhealthwhitepaper.pdf. Accessed July 22, 2020.
50. Ghezzi EM. The development of the Coalition for Oral Health for the Aging. Spec Care Dentist 2011;31(5):147–9.

Moving?

Make sure your subscription moves with you!

To notify us of your new address, find your **Clinics Account Number** (located on your mailing label above your name), and contact customer service at:

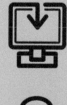

Email: journalscustomerservice-usa@elsevier.com

800-654-2452 (subscribers in the U.S. & Canada)
314-447-8871 (subscribers outside of the U.S. & Canada)

Fax number: 314-447-8029

Elsevier Health Sciences Division
Subscription Customer Service
3251 Riverport Lane
Maryland Heights, MO 63043

*To ensure uninterrupted delivery of your subscription, please notify us at least 4 weeks in advance of move.

Printed and bound by CPI Group (UK) Ltd, Croydon, CR0 4YY

03/10/2024

01040471-0014